THE OFFICIAL PATIENT'S SOURCEBOOK

on

ACANTHAMOEBA INFECTION

JAMES N. PARKER, M.D.
AND PHILIP M. PARKER, PH.D., EDITORS

ICON Health Publications
ICON Group International, Inc.
4370 La Jolla Village Drive, 4th Floor
San Diego, CA 92122 USA

Printed in the United States of America.

Last digit indicates print number: 10 9 8 7 6 4 5 3 2 1

Publisher, Health Care: Tiffany LaRochelle
Editor(s): James Parker, M.D., Philip Parker, Ph.D.

Publisher's note: The ideas, procedures, and suggestions contained in this book are not intended as a substitute for consultation with your physician. All matters regarding your health require medical supervision. As new medical or scientific information becomes available from academic and clinical research, recommended treatments and drug therapies may undergo changes. The authors, editors, and publisher have attempted to make the information in this book up to date and accurate in accord with accepted standards at the time of publication. The authors, editors, and publisher are not responsible for errors or omissions or for consequences from application of the book, and make no warranty, expressed or implied, in regard to the contents of this book. Any practice described in this book should be applied by the reader in accordance with professional standards of care used in regard to the unique circumstances that may apply in each situation, in close consultation with a qualified physician. The reader is advised to always check product information (package inserts) for changes and new information regarding dose and contraindications before taking any drug or pharmacological product. Caution is especially urged when using new or infrequently ordered drugs, herbal remedies, vitamins and supplements, alternative therapies, complementary therapies and medicines, and integrative medical treatments.

Cataloging-in-Publication Data

Parker, James N., 1961-
Parker, Philip M., 1960-

The Official Patient's Sourcebook on Acanthamoeba Infection: A Revised and Updated Directory for the Internet Age/James N. Parker and Philip M. Parker, editors
        p.   cm.
Includes bibliographical references, glossary and index.
ISBN: 0-597-83359-1
1. Acanthamoeba Infection-Popular works.   I. Title.

Disclaimer

This publication is not intended to be used for the diagnosis or treatment of a health problem or as a substitute for consultation with licensed medical professionals. It is sold with the understanding that the publisher, editors, and authors are not engaging in the rendering of medical, psychological, financial, legal, or other professional services.

References to any entity, product, service, or source of information that may be contained in this publication should not be considered an endorsement, either direct or implied, by the publisher, editors or authors. ICON Group International, Inc., the editors, or the authors are not responsible for the content of any Web pages nor publications referenced in this publication.

Copyright Notice

Dedication

To the healthcare professionals dedicating their time and efforts to the study of Acanthamoeba infection.

Acknowledgements

The collective knowledge generated from academic and applied research summarized in various references has been critical in the creation of this sourcebook which is best viewed as a comprehensive compilation and collection of information prepared by various official agencies which directly or indirectly are dedicated to Acanthamoeba infection. All of the *Official Patient's Sourcebooks* draw from various agencies and institutions associated with the United States Department of Health and Human Services, and in particular, the Office of the Secretary of Health and Human Services (OS), the Administration for Children and Families (ACF), the Administration on Aging (AOA), the Agency for Healthcare Research and Quality (AHRQ), the Agency for Toxic Substances and Disease Registry (ATSDR), the Centers for Disease Control and Prevention (CDC), the Food and Drug Administration (FDA), the Healthcare Financing Administration (HCFA), the Health Resources and Services Administration (HRSA), the Indian Health Service (IHS), the institutions of the National Institutes of Health (NIH), the Program Support Center (PSC), and the Substance Abuse and Mental Health Services Administration (SAMHSA). In addition to these sources, information gathered from the National Library of Medicine, the United States Patent Office, the European Union, and their related organizations has been invaluable in the creation of this sourcebook. Some of the work represented was financially supported by the Research and Development Committee at INSEAD. This support is gratefully acknowledged. Finally, special thanks are owed to Tiffany LaRochelle for her excellent editorial support.

v

About the Editors

James N. Parker, M.D.

Dr. James N. Parker received his Bachelor of Science degree in Psychobiology from the University of California, Riverside and his M.D. from the University of California, San Diego. In addition to authoring numerous research publications, he has lectured at various academic institutions. Dr. Parker is the medical editor for the *Official Patient's Sourcebook* series published by ICON Health Publications.

Philip M. Parker, Ph.D.

Philip M. Parker is the Eli Lilly Chair Professor of Innovation, Business and Society at INSEAD (Fontainebleau, France and Singapore). Dr. Parker has also been Professor at the University of California, San Diego and has taught courses at Harvard University, the Hong Kong University of Science and Technology, the Massachusetts Institute of Technology, Stanford University, and UCLA. Dr. Parker is the associate editor for the *Official Patient's Sourcebook* series published by ICON Health Publications.

About ICON Health Publications

In addition to Acanthamoeba infection, *Official Patient's Sourcebooks* are available for the following related topics:

- The Official Patient's Sourcebook on Alveolar Hydatid Disease
- The Official Patient's Sourcebook on Amebiasis
- The Official Patient's Sourcebook on Angiostrongylus Cantonensis
- The Official Patient's Sourcebook on Anisakiasis
- The Official Patient's Sourcebook on Ascaris Infection
- The Official Patient's Sourcebook on Babesia Infection
- The Official Patient's Sourcebook on Balantidiasis
- The Official Patient's Sourcebook on Baylisascaris
- The Official Patient's Sourcebook on Blastocystis Hominis
- The Official Patient's Sourcebook on Body Lice
- The Official Patient's Sourcebook on Capillaria Infection
- The Official Patient's Sourcebook on Chagas Disease
- The Official Patient's Sourcebook on Chronic Diarrhea
- The Official Patient's Sourcebook on Clonorchiasis
- The Official Patient's Sourcebook on Cryptosporidium
- The Official Patient's Sourcebook on Cysticercosis
- The Official Patient's Sourcebook on Dientamoeba Fragilis
- The Official Patient's Sourcebook on Diphyllobothrium Infection
- The Official Patient's Sourcebook on Dipylidium Infection
- The Official Patient's Sourcebook on Dracunculiasis
- The Official Patient's Sourcebook on East African Trypanosomiasis
- The Official Patient's Sourcebook on Fasciola Infection
- The Official Patient's Sourcebook on Fasciolopsiasis
- The Official Patient's Sourcebook on Giardiasis
- The Official Patient's Sourcebook on Gnathostoma Infection
- The Official Patient's Sourcebook on Head Lice
- The Official Patient's Sourcebook on Heterophyes Infection
- The Official Patient's Sourcebook on Hookworm
- The Official Patient's Sourcebook on Hymenloepis Infection
- The Official Patient's Sourcebook on Infection with Nonpathogenic Intestinal Amebas
- The Official Patient's Sourcebook on Isospora Belli
- The Official Patient's Sourcebook on Leishmaniasis
- The Official Patient's Sourcebook on Lymphatic Filariasis
- The Official Patient's Sourcebook on Microsporidiosis

- The Official Patient's Sourcebook on Naegleria
- The Official Patient's Sourcebook on Opisthorchis
- The Official Patient's Sourcebook on Paragonimus
- The Official Patient's Sourcebook on Pinworm Infection
- The Official Patient's Sourcebook on Pneumocystis Carinii
- The Official Patient's Sourcebook on Pubic Lice
- The Official Patient's Sourcebook on Scabies
- The Official Patient's Sourcebook on Schistosomiasis
- The Official Patient's Sourcebook on Strongyloides
- The Official Patient's Sourcebook on Swimmer's Itch
- The Official Patient's Sourcebook on Taenia Saginata
- The Official Patient's Sourcebook on Toxocariasis
- The Official Patient's Sourcebook on Toxoplasmosis
- The Official Patient's Sourcebook on Trichinosis
- The Official Patient's Sourcebook on Trichomonas Infection
- The Official Patient's Sourcebook on Trichuris Trichiura
- The Official Patient's Sourcebook on West African Trypanosomiasis

To discover more about ICON Health Publications, simply check with your preferred online booksellers, including Barnes & Noble.com and Amazon.com which currently carry all of our titles. Or, feel free to contact us directly for bulk purchases or institutional discounts:

ICON Group International, Inc.
4370 La Jolla Village Drive, Fourth Floor
San Diego, CA 92122 USA
Fax: 858-546-4341
Web site: **www.icongrouponline.com/health**

Table of Contents

INTRODUCTION

Overview

Dr. C. Everett Koop, former U.S. Surgeon General, once said, "The best prescription is knowledge."[1] The Agency for Healthcare Research and Quality (AHRQ) of the National Institutes of Health (NIH) echoes this view and recommends that every patient incorporate education into the treatment process. According to the AHRQ:

> Finding out more about your condition is a good place to start. By contacting groups that support your condition, visiting your local library, and searching on the Internet, you can find good information to help guide your treatment decisions. Some information may be hard to find — especially if you don't know where to look.[2]

As the AHRQ mentions, finding the right information is not an obvious task. Though many physicians and public officials had thought that the emergence of the Internet would do much to assist patients in obtaining reliable information, in March 2001 the National Institutes of Health issued the following warning:

> The number of Web sites offering health-related resources grows every day. Many sites provide valuable information, while others may have information that is unreliable or misleading.[3]

---

[1] Quotation from **http://www.drkoop.com**.
[2] The Agency for Healthcare Research and Quality (AHRQ):
http://www.ahcpr.gov/consumer/diaginfo.htm.
[3] From the NIH, National Cancer Institute (NCI):
http://cancertrials.nci.nih.gov/beyond/evaluating.html.

Since the late 1990s, physicians have seen a general increase in patient Internet usage rates. Patients frequently enter their doctor's offices with printed Web pages of home remedies in the guise of latest medical research. This scenario is so common that doctors often spend more time dispelling misleading information than guiding patients through sound therapies. *The Official Patient's Sourcebook on Acanthamoeba Infection* has been created for patients who have decided to make education and research an integral part of the treatment process. The pages that follow will tell you where and how to look for information covering virtually all topics related to Acanthamoeba infection, from the essentials to the most advanced areas of research.

The title of this book includes the word "official." This reflects the fact that the sourcebook draws from public, academic, government, and peer-reviewed research. Selected readings from various agencies are reproduced to give you some of the latest official information available to date on Acanthamoeba infection.

Given patients' increasing sophistication in using the Internet, abundant references to reliable Internet-based resources are provided throughout this sourcebook. Where possible, guidance is provided on how to obtain free-of-charge, primary research results as well as more detailed information via the Internet. E-book and electronic versions of this sourcebook are fully interactive with each of the Internet sites mentioned (clicking on a hyperlink automatically opens your browser to the site indicated). Hard copy users of this sourcebook can type cited Web addresses directly into their browsers to obtain access to the corresponding sites. Since we are working with ICON Health Publications, hard copy *Sourcebooks* are frequently updated and printed on demand to ensure that the information provided is current.

In addition to extensive references accessible via the Internet, every chapter presents a "Vocabulary Builder." Many health guides offer glossaries of technical or uncommon terms in an appendix. In editing this sourcebook, we have decided to place a smaller glossary within each chapter that covers terms used in that chapter. Given the technical nature of some chapters, you may need to revisit many sections. Building one's vocabulary of medical terms in such a gradual manner has been shown to improve the learning process.

We must emphasize that no sourcebook on Acanthamoeba infection should affirm that a specific diagnostic procedure or treatment discussed in a research study, patent, or doctoral dissertation is "correct" or your best option. This sourcebook is no exception. Each patient is unique. Deciding on appropriate options is always up to the patient in consultation with their physician and healthcare providers.

Organization

This sourcebook is organized into three parts. Part I explores basic techniques to researching Acanthamoeba infection (e.g. finding guidelines on diagnosis, treatments, and prognosis), followed by a number of topics, including information on how to get in touch with organizations, associations, or other patient networks dedicated to Acanthamoeba infection. It also gives you sources of information that can help you find a doctor in your local area specializing in treating Acanthamoeba infection. Collectively, the material presented in Part I is a complete primer on basic research topics for patients with Acanthamoeba infection.

Part II moves on to advanced research dedicated to Acanthamoeba infection. Part II is intended for those willing to invest many hours of hard work and study. It is here that we direct you to the latest scientific and applied research on Acanthamoeba infection. When possible, contact names, links via the Internet, and summaries are provided. It is in Part II where the vocabulary process becomes important as authors publishing advanced research frequently use highly specialized language. In general, every attempt is made to recommend "free-to-use" options.

Part III provides appendices of useful background reading for all patients with Acanthamoeba infection or related disorders. The appendices are dedicated to more pragmatic issues faced by many patients with Acanthamoeba infection. Accessing materials via medical libraries may be the only option for some readers, so a guide is provided for finding local medical libraries which are open to the public. Part III, therefore, focuses on advice that goes beyond the biological and scientific issues facing patients with Acanthamoeba infection.

Scope

While this sourcebook covers Acanthamoeba infection, your doctor, research publications, and specialists may refer to your condition using a variety of terms. Therefore, you should understand that Acanthamoeba infection is often considered a synonym or a condition closely related to the following:

- Acanthamoeba Keratitis

- Bacterial Keratitis
- Fungal Keratitis
- Herpes Simplex Keratitis

For the purposes of this sourcebook, we have attempted to be as inclusive as possible, looking for official information for all of the synonyms relevant to Acanthamoeba infection. You may find it useful to refer to synonyms when accessing databases or interacting with healthcare professionals and medical librarians.

Moving Forward

Since the 1980s, the world has seen a proliferation of healthcare guides covering most illnesses. Some are written by patients or their family members. These generally take a layperson's approach to understanding and coping with an illness or disorder. They can be uplifting, encouraging, and highly supportive. Other guides are authored by physicians or other healthcare providers who have a more clinical outlook. Each of these two styles of guide has its purpose and can be quite useful.

As editors, we have chosen a third route. We have chosen to expose you to as many sources of official and peer-reviewed information as practical, for the purpose of educating you about basic and advanced knowledge as recognized by medical science today. You can think of this sourcebook as your personal Internet age reference librarian.

Why "Internet age"? All too often, patients diagnosed with Acanthamoeba infection will log on to the Internet, type words into a search engine, and receive several Web site listings which are mostly irrelevant or redundant. These patients are left to wonder where the relevant information is, and how to obtain it. Since only the smallest fraction of information dealing with Acanthamoeba infection is even indexed in search engines, a non-systematic approach often leads to frustration and disappointment. With this sourcebook, we hope to direct you to the information you need that you would not likely find using popular Web directories. Beyond Web listings, in many cases we will reproduce brief summaries or abstracts of available reference materials. These abstracts often contain distilled information on topics of discussion.

Before beginning your search for information, it is important for you to realize that Acanthamoeba infection is considered a relatively uncommon condition. Because of this, far less research is conducted on Acanthamoeba infection compared to other health problems afflicting larger populations, like breast cancer or heart disease. Nevertheless, this sourcebook will prove useful for two reasons. First, if more information does become available on Acanthamoeba infection, the sources given in this book will be the most likely to report or make such information available. Second, some will find it important to know about patient support, symptom management, or diagnostic procedures that may be relevant to both Acanthamoeba infection and other conditions. By using the sources listed in the following chapters, self-directed research can be conducted on broader topics that are related to Acanthamoeba infection but not readily uncovered using general Internet search engines (e.g. www.google.com or www.yahoo.com). In this way, we have designed this sourcebook to complement these general search engines that can provide useful information and access to online patient support groups.[4]

While we focus on the more scientific aspects of Acanthamoeba infection, there is, of course, the emotional side to consider. Later in the sourcebook, we provide a chapter dedicated to helping you find peer groups and associations that can provide additional support beyond research produced by medical science. We hope that the choices we have made give you the most options available in moving forward. In this way, we wish you the best in your efforts to incorporate this educational approach into your treatment plan.

The Editors

---

[4] For example, one can simply go to **www.google.com,** or other general search engines (e.g. **www.yahoo.com, www.aol.com, www.msn.com**) and type in "Acanthamoeba infection support group" to find any active online support groups dedicated to Acanthamoeba infection.

PART I: THE ESSENTIALS

ABOUT PART I

Part I has been edited to give you access to what we feel are "the essentials" on Acanthamoeba infection. The essentials of a disease typically include the definition or description of the disease, a discussion of who it affects, the signs or symptoms associated with the disease, tests or diagnostic procedures that might be specific to the disease, and treatments for the disease. Your doctor or healthcare provider may have already explained the essentials of Acanthamoeba infection to you or even given you a pamphlet or brochure describing Acanthamoeba infection. Now you are searching for more in-depth information. As editors, we have decided, nevertheless, to include a discussion on where to find essential information that can complement what your doctor has already told you. In this section we recommend a process, not a particular Web site or reference book. The process ensures that, as you search the Web, you gain background information in such a way as to maximize your understanding.

CHAPTER 1. THE ESSENTIALS ON ACANTHAMOEBA INFECTION: GUIDELINES

Overview

Official agencies, as well as federally-funded institutions supported by national grants, frequently publish a variety of guidelines on Acanthamoeba infection. These are typically called "Fact Sheets" or "Guidelines." They can take the form of a brochure, information kit, pamphlet, or flyer. Often they are only a few pages in length. The great advantage of guidelines over other sources is that they are often written with the patient in mind. Since new guidelines on Acanthamoeba infection can appear at any moment and be published by a number of sources, the best approach to finding guidelines is to systematically scan the Internet-based services that post them.

The National Institutes of Health (NIH)[5]

The National Institutes of Health (NIH) is the first place to search for relatively current patient guidelines and fact sheets on Acanthamoeba infection. Originally founded in 1887, the NIH is one of the world's foremost medical research centers and the federal focal point for medical research in the United States. At any given time, the NIH supports some 35,000 research grants at universities, medical schools, and other research and training institutions, both nationally and internationally. The rosters of those who have conducted research or who have received NIH support over the years include the world's most illustrious scientists and physicians. Among them are 97 scientists who have won the Nobel Prize for achievement in medicine.

---

[5] Adapted from the NIH: **http://www.nih.gov/about/NIHoverview.html**.

There is no guarantee that any one Institute will have a guideline on a specific disease, though the National Institutes of Health collectively publish over 600 guidelines for both common and rare diseases. The best way to access NIH guidelines is via the Internet. Although the NIH is organized into many different Institutes and Offices, the following is a list of key Web sites where you are most likely to find NIH clinical guidelines and publications dealing with Acanthamoeba infection and associated conditions:

- Office of the Director (OD); guidelines consolidated across agencies available at **http://www.nih.gov/health/consumer/conkey.htm**

- National Library of Medicine (NLM); extensive encyclopedia (A.D.A.M., Inc.) with guidelines available at **http://www.nlm.nih.gov/medlineplus/healthtopics.html**

- National Institute of Allergy and Infectious Diseases (NIAID); guidelines available at **http://www.niaid.nih.gov/publications/**

- Centers for Disease Control and Prevention: various fact sheets on infectious diseases at **http://www.cdc.gov/health/diseases.htm**

Among the above, the National Institute of Allergy and Infectious Diseases (NIAID) is particularly noteworthy. The mission of the NIAID is to provide support for scientists conducting research aimed at developing better ways to diagnose, treat, and prevent the many infectious, immunologic and allergic diseases that afflict people worldwide.[6] The NIAID is composed of four extramural divisions: the Division of AIDS; the Division of Allergy, Immunology and Transplantation; the Division of Microbiology and Infectious Diseases; and the Division of Extramural Activities. In addition, NIAID scientists conduct intramural research in laboratories located in Bethesda, Rockville and Frederick, Maryland, and in Hamilton, Montana. The following patient guideline was recently published by the NIAID on Acanthamoeba infection.

What Is Acanthamoeba Infection?[7]

Acanthamoeba are microscopic ameba commonly found in the environment. Several species of Acanthamoeba have been found to infect humans, A.

---

[6] This paragraph has been adapted from the NIAID: **http://www.niaid.nih.gov/facts/overview.htm**. "Adapted" signifies that a passage has been reproduced exactly or slightly edited for this book.

[7] Adapted from the Centers for Disease Control and Prevention (CDC): **http://www.cdc.gov/ncidod/dpd/parasites/acanthomoeba/factsht_acanthamoeba.htm**.

culbertsoni, A. polyphaga, A. castellanii, A. healyi, (A. astronyxis), A. hatchetti, A. rhysodes, and possibly others.

Where Are Acanthamoeba Found?

Acanthamoeba spp. (spp. means several species) are found worldwide. Most commonly, Acanthamoeba are found in the soil and dust, in fresh water sources such as lakes, rivers, and hot springs and in hot tubs. Acanthamoeba may also be found in brackish water and in sea water. Amebas can also be found in Heating, Venting, and Air Conditioner units (HVAC), humidifiers, dialysis units, and contact lens paraphernalia.

Acanthamoeba have been found in the nose and throat of healthy people as well as those with compromised immune systems.

How Does Infection with Acanthamoeba Occur?

Acanthamoeba can enter the skin through a cut, wound, or through the nostrils. Once inside the body, amebas can travel to the lungs and through the bloodstream to other parts of the body, especially the central nervous system (brain and spinal cord).

Through improper storage, handling, and disinfection of contact lenses, Acanthamoeba can enter the eye and cause a serious infection.

What Are the Signs and Symptoms of Acanthamoeba Infection?

There are several ways Acanthamoeba spp. can affect the body.

Each year, many people are infected with Acanthamoeba. Eye infections result from contact lens cases becoming contaminated after improper cleaning and handling. Risk of Acanthamoeba infection is higher for people who make their own contact lens cleaning solution. Acanthamoeba enter the eye via contact lenses or through a corneal cut or sore. Infection or a corneal ulcer results.

In addition, Acanthamoeba spp. can cause skin lesions and/or a systemic (whole body) infection. Acanthamoeba spp. cause a serious, most often deadly infection called granulomatous amebic encephalitis (GAE). Once infected, a person may suffer with headaches, stiff neck, nausea and vomiting, tiredness, confusion, lack of attention to people and surroundings, loss of balance and bodily control, seizures, and hallucinations. Signs and symptoms progresses over several weeks; death generally occurs.

Who Is at Risk for Infection with Acanthamoeba?

Infections caused by Acanthamoeba spp. occur more frequently in people with compromised immune systems or those who are chronically ill.

Is There Treatment for Infection with Acanthamoeba?

Yes. Eye and skin infections are generally treatable. Although most cases of brain (CNS) infection with Acanthamoeba have been fatal, a few however, have recovered from the infection with proper treatment. Acanthamoeba infections of the brain (CNS) are almost always fatal.

Can Infection Be Spread from Person to Person?

No cases have ever been reported.

How Can I Prevent an Infection with Acanthamoeba?

Eye infections may be prevented by using commercially prepared contact lens cleaning solution rather than making and using home-made solutions. There is little that can be done to prevent skin and body infection.

For More Information

- Centers for Disease Control. Acanthamoeba keratitis associated with contact lenses–United States. MMWR 1986:35: 405-8.
- Centers for Disease Control. Acanthamoeba keratitis associated with soft contact lens wearers–United States. MMWR 1987; 36:397-8, 403-4.
- Ma P, Visvesvara GS, Martinez AJ, Theodore FH, Daggett PM, Sawyer TK. Naegleria and Acanthamoeba infections: Review. Rev Infect Dis 1990; 12:490-513.

- Visvesvara GS, Stehr-Green JK. Epidemiology of free-living ameba infections. J Protozool 1990; 37:25S-33S.

- Martinez AJ, Visvesvara GS. Free-living, amphizoic and opportunistic amebas. Brain Pathol 1997; 7:583-598.

Acanthamoeba Infection: Technical Notes

DPDx is a Web site developed and maintained by CDC's Division of Parasitic Diseases (DPD). Their goal is to use the internet to strengthen diagnosis of parasitic diseases, both in the United States and abroad. For that purpose, DPDx offers two complementary functions: (1) a reference and training function, in which all users can browse through concise reviews of parasites and parasitic diseases, including an image library and a review of recommended procedures for collecting, shipping, processing, and examining biologic specimens, and (2) a diagnostic assistance function, in which laboratorians and other health professionals desiring assistance in parasite identification can ask questions and/or send digital images of specimens for expedited review and consultation with DPD staff. The review below is adapted from a DPDx review of Acanthamoeba infection.[8] As the information was prepared for healthcare professionals, some of the language is technical. Relevant terms are defined in the glossary builder at the end of this chapter.

Causal Agents

Naegleria fowleri and Acanthamoeba spp., commonly found in lakes, swimming pools, tap water, and heating and air conditioning units. While only one species of Naegleria is known to infect humans, several species of Acanthamoeba are implicated, including A. culbertsoni, A. polyphaga, A. castellanii, A. astronyxis, A. hatchetti, and A. rhysodes. An additional agent of human disease, Balamuthia mandrillaris, is a related leptomyxid ameba that is morphologically similar in light microscopy to Acanthamoeba.

---

[8] This paragraph has been adapted from the DPDx:
http://www.dpd.cdc.gov/dpdx/HTML/FreeLivingAmebic.htm.
The review of Acanthamoeba infection has been adapted from the DPDx Web site. Further treatment information in The Medical Letter (http://www.medletter.com/) is recommended by the DPDx. The section of "Diagnostic Findings" which provides diagnostic images and related information should be viewed separately at: http://www.dpd.cdc.gov/dpdx/HTML/Frames/A-F/FreeLivingAmebic/body_FreeLivingAmebic_mic1.htm .

Life Cycle

Naegleria fowleri is found in nature in warm water bodies as ameboid and ameboflagellate trophozoites. Cysts also occur in nature, but not in human infections. Infection occurs during swimming or diving with the parasites gaining access, through the olfactory neuroepithelium, to the brain. Acanthamoeba spp. occur in the same environments, but are also found in soil and dust as well as more restricted liquid environments such as humidifiers and dialysis units. (They can also be cultured from the upper respiratory tract of some healthy individuals.) Acanthamoeba spp. do not have an ameboflagellate form, and cysts can be found in human infections. Infections due to Acanthamoeba spp. occur more frequently in debilitated or chronically ill individuals, and reach the central nervous system by hematogenous dissemination from foci in the lungs, skin, or sinuses.

Geographic Distribution

While infrequent, infections appear to occur worldwide.

Clinical Features

Acute primary amebic meningoencephalitis (PAM) is caused by Naegleria fowleri. It presents with severe headache and other meningeal signs, fever, vomiting, and focal neurologic deficits, and progresses rapidly (<10 days) and frequently to coma and death. Acanthamoeba spp. causes mostly subacute or chronic granulomatous amebic encephalitis (GAE), with a clinical picture of headaches, altered mental status, and focal neurologic deficit, which progresses over several weeks to death. In addition, Acanthamoeba spp. can cause granulomatous skin lesions and, more seriously, keratitis and corneal ulcers following corneal trauma or in association with contact lenses.

Laboratory Diagnosis

In Naegleria infections, the diagnosis can be made by microscopic examination of cerebrospinal fluid (CSF). A wet mount may detect motile trophozoites, and a Giemsa-stained smear will show trophozoites with typical morphology. In Acanthamoeba infections, the diagnosis can be made from microscopic examination of stained smears of biopsy specimens (brain tissue, skin, cornea) or of corneal scrapings, which may detect trophozoites and cysts. Cultivation of the causal organism, and its identification by direct immunofluorescent antibody, may also prove useful.

Treatment

Eye and skin infections caused by Acanthamoeba spp. are generally treatable. Topical use of 0.1% propamidine isethionate (Brolene) plus neomycin-polymyxin B-gramicidin ophthalmic solution has been a successful approach; keratoplasty is often necessary in severe infections. Although most cases of brain (CNS) infection with Acanthamoeba have resulted in death, patients have recovered from the infection with proper treatment.

More Guideline Sources

The guideline above on Acanthamoeba infection is only one example of the kind of material that you can find online and free of charge. The remainder of this chapter will direct you to other sources which either publish or can help you find additional guidelines on topics related to Acanthamoeba infection. Many of the guidelines listed below address topics that may be of particular relevance to your specific situation or of special interest to only some patients with Acanthamoeba infection. Due to space limitations these sources are listed in a concise manner. Do not hesitate to consult the following sources by either using the Internet hyperlink provided, or, in cases where the contact information is provided, contacting the publisher or author directly.

Topic Pages: MEDLINEplus

For patients wishing to go beyond guidelines published by specific Institutes of the NIH, the National Library of Medicine has created a vast and patient-oriented healthcare information portal called MEDLINEplus. Within this Internet-based system are "health topic pages." You can think of a health topic page as a guide to patient guides. To access this system, log on to **http://www.nlm.nih.gov/medlineplus/healthtopics.html**. From there you can either search using the alphabetical index or browse by broad topic areas.

If you do not find topics of interest when browsing health topic pages, then you can choose to use the advanced search utility of MEDLINEplus at **http://www.nlm.nih.gov/medlineplus/advancedsearch.html**. This utility is similar to the NIH Search Utility, with the exception that it only includes material linked within the MEDLINEplus system (mostly patient-oriented information). It also has the disadvantage of generating unstructured results. We recommend, therefore, that you use this method only if you have a very targeted search.

The National Guideline Clearinghouse™

The National Guideline Clearinghouse™ offers hundreds of evidence-based clinical practice guidelines published in the United States and other countries. You can search their site located at **http://www.guideline.gov** by using the keyword "Acanthamoeba infection" or synonyms. The following was recently posted:

- **Care of the contact lens patient.**

  Source: American Optometric Association.; 2000; 77 pages

  http://www.guideline.gov/FRAMESETS/guideline_fs.asp?guideline=001829&sSearch_string=acanthamoeba+infection

- **Refractive errors.**

  Source: American Academy of Ophthalmology.; 1997 September; 38 pages

  http://www.guideline.gov/FRAMESETS/guideline_fs.asp?guideline=000411&sSearch_string=acanthamoeba+infection

Healthfinder™

Healthfinder™ is an additional source sponsored by the U.S. Department of Health and Human Services which offers links to hundreds of other sites that contain healthcare information. This Web site is located at **http://www.healthfinder.gov**. Again, keyword searches can be used to find guidelines.

The NIH Search Utility

After browsing the references listed at the beginning of this chapter, you may want to explore the NIH Search Utility. This allows you to search for documents on over 100 selected Web sites that comprise the NIH-WEB-SPACE. Each of these servers is "crawled" and indexed on an ongoing basis. Your search will produce a list of various documents, all of which will relate in some way to Acanthamoeba infection. The drawbacks of this approach are that the information is not organized by theme and that the references are often a mix of information for professionals and patients. Nevertheless, a large number of the listed Web sites provide useful background information. We can only recommend this route, therefore, for relatively rare or specific disorders, or when using highly targeted searches. To use the NIH search utility, visit the following Web page: **http://search.nih.gov/index.html**.

Additional Web Sources

A number of Web sites that often link to government sites are available to the public. These can also point you in the direction of essential information. The following is a representative sample:

- AOL: **http://search.aol.com/cat.adp?id=168&layer=&from=subcats**

- drkoop.com®: **http://www.drkoop.com/conditions/ency/index.html**

- Family Village: **http://www.familyvillage.wisc.edu/specific.htm**

- Google: **http://directory.google.com/Top/Health/Conditions_and_Diseases/**

- Med Help International: **http://www.medhelp.org/HealthTopics/A.html**

- Open Directory Project: **http://dmoz.org/Health/Conditions_and_Diseases/**

- Yahoo.com: **http://dir.yahoo.com/Health/Diseases_and_Conditions/**

- WebMD®Health: **http://my.webmd.com/health_topics**

Vocabulary Builder

The material in this chapter may have contained a number of unfamiliar words. The following Vocabulary Builder introduces you to terms used in this chapter that have not been covered in the previous chapter:

Acanthamoeba: A genus of free-living soil amoebae that produces no flagellate stage. Its organisms are pathogens for several infections in humans and have been found in the eye, bone, brain, and respiratory tract. [NIH]

Antibody: An immunoglobulin molecule that has a specific amino acid sequence by virtue of which it interacts only with the antigen that induced its synthesis in cells of the lymphoid series (especially plasma cells), or with antigen closely related to it. Antibodies are classified according to their ode of action as agglutinins, bacteriolysins, haemolysins, opsonins, precipitins, etc. [EU]

Biopsy: The removal and examination, usually microscopic, of tissue from the living body, performed to establish precise diagnosis. [EU]

Causal: Pertaining to a cause; directed against a cause. [EU]

Cerebrospinal: Pertaining to the brain and spinal cord. [EU]

Cyst: Any closed cavity or sac; normal or abnormal, lined by epithelium, and especially one that contains a liquid or semisolid material. [EU]

Disinfection: Rendering pathogens harmless through the use of heat, antiseptics, antibacterial agents, etc. [NIH]

Diving: An activity in which the organism plunges into water. It includes scuba and bell diving. Diving as natural behavior of animals goes here, as well as diving in decompression experiments with humans or animals. [NIH]

Encephalitis: Inflammation of the brain. [EU]

Fatal: Causing death, deadly; mortal; lethal. [EU]

Gramicidin: Antibiotic mixture that is one of the two principle components of tyrothricin from Bacillus brevis. Gramicidin C or S is a cyclic, ten-amino acid polypeptide and gramicidins A, B, D, etc., seem to be linear polypeptides. The mixture is used topically for gram-positive organisms. It is toxic to blood, liver, kidneys, meninges, and the olfactory apparatus. [NIH]

Keratitis: Inflammation of the cornea. [EU]

Lenses: Pieces of glass or other transparent materials used for magnification or increased visual acuity. [NIH]

Lesion: Any pathological or traumatic discontinuity of tissue or loss of function of a part. [EU]

Mental: Pertaining to the mind; psychic. 2. (L. mentum chin) pertaining to the chin. [EU]

Microbiology: The study of microorganisms such as fungi, bacteria, algae, archaea, and viruses. [NIH]

Microscopy: The application of microscope magnification to the study of materials that cannot be properly seen by the unaided eye. [NIH]

Naegleria: A free-living soil amoeba pathogenic to humans and animals. It occurs also in water and sewage. The most commonly found species in man is naegleri fowleri which is the pathogen for primary amebic meningoencephalitis in primates. [NIH]

Nausea: An unpleasant sensation, vaguely referred to the epigastrium and abdomen, and often culminating in vomiting. [EU]

Neomycin: Antibiotic complex produced by Streptomyces fradiae. It is composed of neomycins A, B, and C. It acts by inhibiting translation during protein synthesis. [NIH]

Neurologic: Pertaining to neurology or to the nervous system. [EU]

Ophthalmic: Pertaining to the eye. [EU]

Ophthalmology: A surgical specialty concerned with the structure and function of the eye and the medical and surgical treatment of its defects and diseases. [NIH]

Polymyxin: Basic polypeptide antibiotic group obtained from Bacillus polymyxa. They affect the cell membrane by detergent action and may cause neuromuscular and kidney damage. At least eleven different members of the polymyxin group have been identified, each designated by a letter. [NIH]

Seizures: Clinical or subclinical disturbances of cortical function due to a sudden, abnormal, excessive, and disorganized discharge of brain cells. Clinical manifestations include abnormal motor, sensory and psychic phenomena. Recurrent seizures are usually referred to as epilepsy or "seizure disorder." [NIH]

Species: A taxonomic category subordinate to a genus (or subgenus) and superior to a subspecies or variety, composed of individuals possessing common characters distinguishing them from other categories of individuals of the same taxonomic level. In taxonomic nomenclature, species are designated by the genus name followed by a Latin or Latinized adjective or noun. [EU]

Subacute: Somewhat acute; between acute and chronic. [EU]

Topical: Pertaining to a particular surface area, as a topical anti-infective applied to a certain area of the skin and affecting only the area to which it is applied. [EU]

Ulcer: A local defect, or excavation, of the surface of an organ or tissue; which is produced by the sloughing of inflammatory necrotic tissue. [EU]

Urinary: Pertaining to the urine; containing or secreting urine. [EU]

Venereal: Pertaining or related to or transmitted by sexual contact. [EU]

CHAPTER 2. SEEKING GUIDANCE

Overview

Some patients are comforted by the knowledge that a number of organizations dedicate their resources to helping people with Acanthamoeba infection. These associations can become invaluable sources of information and advice. Many associations offer aftercare support, financial assistance, and other important services. Furthermore, healthcare research has shown that support groups often help people to better cope with their conditions.[9] In addition to support groups, your physician can be a valuable source of guidance and support. Therefore, finding a physician that can work with your unique situation is a very important aspect of your care.

In this chapter, we direct you to resources that can help you find patient organizations and medical specialists. We begin by describing how to find associations and peer groups that can help you better understand and cope with Acanthamoeba infection. The chapter ends with a discussion on how to find a doctor that is right for you.

Associations and Acanthamoeba Infection

As mentioned by the Agency for Healthcare Research and Quality, sometimes the emotional side of an illness can be as taxing as the physical side.[10] You may have fears or feel overwhelmed by your situation. Everyone has different ways of dealing with disease or physical injury. Your attitude, your expectations, and how well you cope with your condition can all

---

[9] Churches, synagogues, and other houses of worship might also have groups that can offer you the social support you need.

[10] This section has been adapted from **http://www.ahcpr.gov/consumer/diaginf5.htm**.

influence your well-being. This is true for both minor conditions and serious illnesses. For example, a study on female breast cancer survivors revealed that women who participated in support groups lived longer and experienced better quality of life when compared with women who did not participate. In the support group, women learned coping skills and had the opportunity to share their feelings with other women in the same situation. There are a number of directories that list additional medical associations that you may find useful. While not all of these directories will provide different information, by consulting all of them, you will have nearly exhausted all sources for patient associations.

The National Health Information Center (NHIC)

The National Health Information Center (NHIC) offers a free referral service to help people find organizations that provide information about Acanthamoeba infection. For more information, see the NHIC's Web site at **http://www.health.gov/NHIC/** or contact an information specialist by calling 1-800-336-4797.

DIRLINE

A comprehensive source of information on associations is the DIRLINE database maintained by the National Library of Medicine. The database comprises some 10,000 records of organizations, research centers, and government institutes and associations which primarily focus on health and biomedicine. DIRLINE is available via the Internet at the following Web site: **http://dirline.nlm.nih.gov/**. Simply type in "Acanthamoeba infection" (or a synonym) or the name of a topic, and the site will list information contained in the database on all relevant organizations.

The Combined Health Information Database

Another comprehensive source of information on healthcare associations is the Combined Health Information Database. Using the "Detailed Search" option, you will need to limit your search to "Organizations" and "Acanthamoeba infection". Type the following hyperlink into your Web browser: **http://chid.nih.gov/detail/detail.html**. To find associations, use the drop boxes at the bottom of the search page where "You may refine your search by." For publication date, select "All Years." Then, select your preferred language and the format option "Organization Resource Sheet." By making these selections and typing in "Acanthamoeba infection" (or synonyms) into the "For these words:" box, you will only receive results on organizations dealing with Acanthamoeba infection. You should check back periodically with this database since it is updated every 3 months.

The National Organization for Rare Disorders, Inc.

The National Organization for Rare Disorders, Inc. has prepared a Web site that provides, at no charge, lists of associations organized by specific diseases. You can access this database at the following Web site: **http://www.rarediseases.org/cgi-bin/nord/searchpage**. Select the option called "Organizational Database (ODB)" and type "Acanthamoeba infection" (or a synonym) in the search box.

Online Support Groups

In addition to support groups, commercial Internet service providers offer forums and chat rooms for people with different illnesses and conditions. WebMD®, for example, offers such a service at their Web site: **http://boards.webmd.com/roundtable**. These online self-help communities can help you connect with a network of people whose concerns are similar to yours. Online support groups are places where people can talk informally. If you read about a novel approach, consult with your doctor or other healthcare providers, as the treatments or discoveries you hear about may not be scientifically proven to be safe and effective.

Finding Doctors

One of the most important aspects of your treatment will be the relationship between you and your doctor or specialist. All patients with Acanthamoeba infection must go through the process of selecting a physician. While this process will vary from person to person, the Agency for Healthcare Research and Quality makes a number of suggestions, including the following:[11]

- If you are in a managed care plan, check the plan's list of doctors first.

- Ask doctors or other health professionals who work with doctors, such as hospital nurses, for referrals.

---

[11] This section is adapted from the AHRQ: **www.ahrq.gov/consumer/qntascii/qntdr.htm** .

- Call a hospital's doctor referral service, but keep in mind that these services usually refer you to doctors on staff at that particular hospital. The services do not have information on the quality of care that these doctors provide.

- Some local medical societies offer lists of member doctors. Again, these lists do not have information on the quality of care that these doctors provide.

Additional steps you can take to locate doctors include the following:

- Check with the associations listed earlier in this chapter.

- Information on doctors in some states is available on the Internet at **http://www.docboard.org**. This Web site is run by "Administrators in Medicine," a group of state medical board directors.

- The American Board of Medical Specialties can tell you if your doctor is board certified. "Certified" means that the doctor has completed a training program in a specialty and has passed an exam, or "board," to assess his or her knowledge, skills, and experience to provide quality patient care in that specialty. Primary care doctors may also be certified as specialists. The AMBS Web site is located at **http://www.abms.org/newsearch.asp**.[12] You can also contact the ABMS by phone at 1-866-ASK-ABMS.

- You can call the American Medical Association (AMA) at 800-665-2882 for information on training, specialties, and board certification for many licensed doctors in the United States. This information also can be found in "Physician Select" at the AMA's Web site: **http://www.ama-assn.org/aps/amahg.htm**.

If the previous sources did not meet your needs, you may want to log on to the Web site of the National Organization for Rare Disorders (NORD) at **http://www.rarediseases.org/**. NORD maintains a database of doctors with expertise in various rare diseases. The Metabolic Information Network (MIN), 800-945-2188, also maintains a database of physicians with expertise in various metabolic diseases.

---

[12] While board certification is a good measure of a doctor's knowledge, it is possible to receive quality care from doctors who are not board certified.

Selecting Your Doctor[3]

When you have compiled a list of prospective doctors, call each of their offices. First, ask if the doctor accepts your health insurance plan and if he or she is taking new patients. If the doctor is not covered by your plan, ask yourself if you are prepared to pay the extra costs. The next step is to schedule a visit with your chosen physician. During the first visit you will have the opportunity to evaluate your doctor and to find out if you feel comfortable with him or her. Ask yourself, did the doctor:

- Give me a chance to ask questions about Acanthamoeba infection?

- Really listen to my questions?

- Answer in terms I understood?

- Show respect for me?

- Ask me questions?

- Make me feel comfortable?

- Address the health problem(s) I came with?

- Ask me my preferences about different kinds of treatments for Acanthamoeba infection?

- Spend enough time with me?

Trust your instincts when deciding if the doctor is right for you. But remember, it might take time for the relationship to develop. It takes more than one visit for you and your doctor to get to know each other.

Working with Your Doctor[4]

Research has shown that patients who have good relationships with their doctors tend to be more satisfied with their care and have better results. Here are some tips to help you and your doctor become partners:

- You know important things about your symptoms and your health history. Tell your doctor what you think he or she needs to know.

- It is important to tell your doctor personal information, even if it makes you feel embarrassed or uncomfortable.

---

[13] This section has been adapted from the AHRQ: **www.ahrq.gov/consumer/qntascii/qntdr.htm**.

[14] This section has been adapted from the AHRQ: **www.ahrq.gov/consumer/qntascii/qntdr.htm**.

- Bring a "health history" list with you (and keep it up to date).

- Always bring any medications you are currently taking with you to the appointment, or you can bring a list of your medications including dosage and frequency information. Talk about any allergies or reactions you have had to your medications.

- Tell your doctor about any natural or alternative medicines you are taking.

- Bring other medical information, such as x-ray films, test results, and medical records.

- Ask questions. If you don't, your doctor will assume that you understood everything that was said.

- Write down your questions before your visit. List the most important ones first to make sure that they are addressed.

- Consider bringing a friend with you to the appointment to help you ask questions. This person can also help you understand and/or remember the answers.

- Ask your doctor to draw pictures if you think that this would help you understand.

- Take notes. Some doctors do not mind if you bring a tape recorder to help you remember things, but always ask first.

- Let your doctor know if you need more time. If there is not time that day, perhaps you can speak to a nurse or physician assistant on staff or schedule a telephone appointment.

- Take information home. Ask for written instructions. Your doctor may also have brochures and audio and videotapes that can help you.

- After leaving the doctor's office, take responsibility for your care. If you have questions, call. If your symptoms get worse or if you have problems with your medication, call. If you had tests and do not hear from your doctor, call for your test results. If your doctor recommended that you have certain tests, schedule an appointment to get them done. If your doctor said you should see an additional specialist, make an appointment.

By following these steps, you will enhance the relationship you will have with your physician.

Broader Health-Related Resources

In addition to the references above, the NIH has set up guidance Web sites that can help patients find healthcare professionals. These include:[15]

- Caregivers:
  http://www.nlm.nih.gov/medlineplus/caregivers.html

- Choosing a Doctor or Healthcare Service:
  http://www.nlm.nih.gov/medlineplus/choosingadoctororhealthcareserv ice.html

- Hospitals and Health Facilities:
  http://www.nlm.nih.gov/medlineplus/healthfacilities.html

---

[15] You can access this information at:
http://www.nlm.nih.gov/medlineplus/healthsystem.html.

PART II: ADDITIONAL RESOURCES AND ADVANCED MATERIAL

ABOUT PART II

In Part II, we introduce you to additional resources and advanced research on Acanthamoeba infection. All too often, patients who conduct their own research are overwhelmed by the difficulty in finding and organizing information. The purpose of the following chapters is to provide you an organized and structured format to help you find additional information resources on Acanthamoeba infection. In Part II, as in Part I, our objective is not to interpret the latest advances on Acanthamoeba infection or render an opinion. Rather, our goal is to give you access to original research and to increase your awareness of sources you may not have already considered. In this way, you will come across the advanced materials often referred to in pamphlets, books, or other general works. Once again, some of this material is technical in nature, so consultation with a professional familiar with Acanthamoeba infection is suggested.

CHAPTER 3. STUDIES ON ACANTHAMOEBA INFECTION

Overview

Every year, academic studies are published on Acanthamoeba infection or related conditions. Broadly speaking, there are two types of studies. The first are peer reviewed. Generally, the content of these studies has been reviewed by scientists or physicians. Peer-reviewed studies are typically published in scientific journals and are usually available at medical libraries. The second type of studies is non-peer reviewed. These works include summary articles that do not use or report scientific results. These often appear in the popular press, newsletters, or similar periodicals.

In this chapter, we will show you how to locate peer-reviewed references and studies on Acanthamoeba infection. We will begin by discussing research that has been summarized and is free to view by the public via the Internet. We then show you how to generate a bibliography on Acanthamoeba infection and teach you how to keep current on new studies as they are published or undertaken by the scientific community.

Federally-Funded Research on Acanthamoeba Infection

The U.S. Government supports a variety of research studies relating to Acanthamoeba infection and associated conditions. These studies are tracked by the Office of Extramural Research at the National Institutes of Health.[16]

---

[16] Healthcare projects are funded by the National Institutes of Health (NIH), Substance Abuse and Mental Health Services (SAMHSA), Health Resources and Services Administration (HRSA), Food and Drug Administration (FDA), Centers for Disease Control

CRISP (Computerized Retrieval of Information on Scientific Projects) is a searchable database of federally-funded biomedical research projects conducted at universities, hospitals, and other institutions. Visit the CRISP Web site at **http://commons.cit.nih.gov/crisp3/CRISP.Generate_Ticket**. You can perform targeted searches by various criteria including geography, date, as well as topics related to Acanthamoeba infection and related conditions.

For most of the studies, the agencies reporting into CRISP provide summaries or abstracts. As opposed to clinical trial research using patients, many federally-funded studies use animals or simulated models to explore Acanthamoeba infection and related conditions. In some cases, therefore, it may be difficult to understand how some basic or fundamental research could eventually translate into medical practice. The following sample is typical of the type of information found when searching the CRISP database for Acanthamoeba infection:

- **Project Title: Anti-Acanthamoeba Eye Infection Drops**

  Principal Investigator & Institution: Smith, Francis X.; Bio-Concept Laboratories, Inc. 4 Tinkham Ave, Ste 104 Derry, Nh 03079

  Timing: Fiscal Year 2000; Project Start 1-MAY-2000; Project End 1-OCT-2000

  Summary: The objective of this project is to develop an eye drop which is more effective than other existing therapies in treating Acanthamoeba keratitis. While a relatively uncommon type of corneal infection, Acanthamoeba keratitis is painfully debilitating and vision-threatening. It is extremely difficult to treat, and the consequences of failure are severe. There is currently no FDA-approved treatment for Acanthamoeba keratitis. Off- label use of various disinfecting agents and antibiotics has provided moderately successful therapy. However, the optimal drug combinations and concentrations and safety of use are not well defined. Bio-Concept Laboratories intends to develop and obtain FDA-approval for a combination of drugs which will be safe and effective. During Phase I of the SBIR funding period, experimental formulations suitable for use on the eye were developed and tested against Acanthamoeba in two distinct in vitro systems. The results showed the ability of the test solutions to kill Acanthamoeba, prevent the cytopathic effect of the parasite in vitro, and give an indication of the optimal concentrations of drug required for therapeutic use. During Phase II, this formulation will be tested in animal models for Acanthamoeba keratitis. The disease will be induced in Chinese hamsters and pigs, and the effectiveness of drug

and Prevention (CDCP), Agency for Healthcare Research and Quality (AHRQ), and Office of Assistant Secretary of Health (OASH).

treatment will be tested against untreated control animals with the disease. Once an effective concentration is determined in the animal model, ophthalmic safety parameters will be established by conducting regulated toxicology studies. Synthesis of the active ingredient will also be required, since it will no longer be available for health care use. Manufacturing procedures and method validation will be conducted as required for sumission to the FDA under an Investigative New Drug application. Proposed Commercial Application: Although the incidence of Acanthamoeba infection is relatively low, there is currently no FDA-approved method for treatment. Thus the Bio-Concept product could capture a major portion of the market. Furthermore, our product has the potential for a broader application which would be effective in treating other ocular microbial infections, substantially increasing potential market value.

Website: http://commons.cit.nih.gov/crisp3/CRISP.Generate_Ticket

- **Project Title: Microglia in Cannabinoid Increased Infectivity**

Principal Investigator & Institution: Marciano-Cabral, Francine; Professor; Virginia Commonwealth University 901 W Franklin St Richmond, Va 23284

Timing: Fiscal Year 2001; Project Start 0-SEP-1988; Project End 1-JUL-2006

Summary: The goal of this study is to define the role of microglia in cannabinoid- mediated increased infectivity of the brain. Microglia, a resident population of macrophages in the brain, respond to trauma and infection by migrating to sites of injury, produce pro-inflammatory cytokines and cytotoxic substances and phagocytize infectious agents and damaged tissues. These cells, also, have been implicated in neuropathological processes such as AIDS dementia and multiple sclerosis. Using a mouse infectivity model we have determined that animals treated with THC and infected with Acanthamoeba, the causative agent of granulomatous amebic encephalitis a chronic disease of the central nervous system, suffer from higher mortalities than do similarly infected vehicle-treated controls. Exacerbated diseased occurred concurrently with dysfunction in microglial responses to infection implicating these cells as targets of THC. We will employ the mouse infectivity model to define the mechanisms by which cannabinoids alter microglial anti-ameba activities to obtain fundamental insight regarding the effects of cannabinoids of microglial resistance to infection of the brain. The hypothesis to be tested is that the exogenous cannabinoid, THC, alters the anti-microbial activities of the microglial cells in response to Acanthamoeba infection which leads to exacerbation of disease. In order to address the hypothesis we will first determine the range of dose responsiveness over which THC inhibits microglial cell functions. We will establish the dose-related THC inhibition of microglial cell migration in relation to time course of infection. In vivo infectivity studies will be complemented with those using in vitro models of microglial migration to Acanthamoeba. Second, we will determine whether THC alters chemotaxis or chemotaxis or purified microglia to Acanthamoeba to Acanthamoeba, to its soluble products, or to cytokines. In addition we will assess whether THC inhibits phagocytosis or amebae or alters effector cell: target cell contact dependent cytotoxicity. Third, we will define the effect of THC on the cytokine expression by immune cells in the brain. Brains from cannabinoid-treated and untreated Acanthamoeba-infected mice will be examined for the production of IL-1, IL-6, IL-10, IL-12, TNF-a, TGF-b, and MIF. Immunological/molecular approaches will be used to establish whether altered expression is effected at the transcriptional, translational, or post-translational levels. Fourth, we will determine the functional relevance of cannabinoid receptors on cannabinoid-mediated altered microglial responsiveness to Acanthamoeba. Stereospecific paired enantiometers, receptor subtype-specific antagonists, , and receptor subtype-specific antibodies, will be employed to determined whether microglial anti-ameba activities are linked to a cannabinoid receptor. Collectively, these studies will allow for definition of the mechanism(s) by which cannabinoids alter resistance to Acanthamoeba and provide valuable insight regarding fundamental processing by which cannabinoids affect brain microglial responses to infectious agents.

Website: http://commons.cit.nih.gov/crisp3/CRISP.Generate_Ticket

- **Project Title: New Treatment for Amoebic Keratitis**

  Principal Investigator & Institution: Villemez, Clarence L.; Molecular Biology; University of Wyoming Box 3355, University Station Laramie, Wy 82071

  Timing: Fiscal Year 2000; Project Start 1-JUL-1999; Project End 0-JUN-2002

  Summary: (Adapted from the applicant's abstract): Acanthamoebic keratitis is an infection of the cornea that is sight threatening. The infective organisms are widely distributed in the United States environment, but are relatively ineffective pathogens. Unlike disseminated Acanthamoeba infections, which are life threatening and occur in patients with compromised immune systems, acanthamoebic keratitis patients appear to be otherwise healthy. Contact lenses appear to increase the probability of contracting the infection. Existing treatment is not sufficiently effective. Even in those cases successfully treated, the disease course is excessively prolonged and involves much pain and loss of vision. This research will investigate the characteristic of Acanthamoeba that appears to determine its opportunistic pathogen property with the aim of developing new therapies. The life cycle of Acanthamoeba, like many important pathogens, includes a dormant form. The putative receptors with which spores and cysts must maintain communication with the extracellular environment are natural focus points for disease prophylaxis and treatment. Yet, except for what is described here, no other receptor of this type has been identified, even from the most studied systems, bacterial spore germination. They have identified a receptor, ESP, which controls absolutely the encystment and excystment of Acanthamoeba castellanii and, consequently, cell division. They also possess four monoclonal antibodies, which react with different epitopes of ESP. Synergy experimentation suggests that ESP is an osmolarity monitor. Anti-ESP bivalent antibodies mimic the natural stimulus for differentiation, causing the organism to cease dividing. The latter characteristic is apparently why Acanthamoeba are poor pathogens. Exploiting this circumstance should easily provide quick and effective therapies for Acanthamoeba pathologies. Experiments will be prepared to extend the ESP/osmolarity receptor results to acanthamoebic keratitis pathogens. They will isolate and sequence the ESP gene from Acanthamoeba castellanii. With polynucleotide probes prepared using the latter information, they will first identify, then isolate, sequence, and employ the homologous genes from pathogenic strains of Acanthamoeba to obtain reasonable quantities of ESP homologs. These proteins, anti-ESP antibodies, and should it prove advantageous, portions of the cDNA, will be used to confer therapeutic immunity. The therapeutic testing will employ the excellent animal models of acanthamoebic keratitis at the University of Texas Southwestern Medical Center, Dallas and the in vivo experiments will be done there.

Website: http://commons.cit.nih.gov/crisp3/CRISP.Generate_Ticket

E-Journals: PubMed Central[17]

PubMed Central (PMC) is a digital archive of life sciences journal literature developed and managed by the National Center for Biotechnology Information (NCBI) at the U.S. National Library of Medicine (NLM).[18] Access

---

[17] Adapted from the National Library of Medicine:
http://www.pubmedcentral.nih.gov/about/intro.html.
[18] With PubMed Central, NCBI is taking the lead in preservation and maintenance of open access to electronic literature, just as NLM has done for decades with printed biomedical literature. PubMed Central aims to become a world-class library of the digital age.

to this growing archive of e-journals is free and unrestricted.[19] To search, go to **http://www.pubmedcentral.nih.gov/index.html#search**, and type "Acanthamoeba infection" (or synonyms) into the search box. This search gives you access to full-text articles. The following is a sample of items found for Acanthamoeba infection in the PubMed Central database:

- **Discrimination between Clinically Relevant and Nonrelevant Acanthamoeba Strains Isolated from Contact Lens- Wearing Keratitis Patients in Austria** by J. Walochnik, E.-M. Haller-Schober, H. Kolli, O. Picher, A. Obwaller, and H. Aspock; 2000 November
  http://www.pubmedcentral.nih.gov/articlerender.fcgi?artid=87520&rendertype=external

- **Granulomatous Amebic Encephalitis in a Patient with AIDS: Isolation of Acanthamoeba sp. Group II from Brain Tissue and Successful Treatment with Sulfadiazine and Fluconazole** by M. Seijo Martinez, G. Gonzalez-Mediero, P. Santiago, A. Rodriguez de Lope, J. Diz, C. Conde, and G. S. Visvesvara; 2000 October
  http://www.pubmedcentral.nih.gov/articlerender.fcgi?artid=87504&rendertype=external

- **Proteases as Markers for Differentiation of Pathogenic and Nonpathogenic Species of Acanthamoeba** by Naveed A. Khan, Edward L. Jarroll, Noorjahan Panjwani, Zhiyi Cao, and Timothy A. Paget; 2000 August
  http://www.pubmedcentral.nih.gov/articlerender.fcgi?artid=87129&rendertype=external

- **Unusual Case of Acanthamoeba polyphaga and Pseudomonas aeruginosa Keratitis in a Contact Lens Wearer from Gauteng, South Africa** by L. A. Dini, C. Cockinos, J. A. Frean, I. A. Niszl, and M. B. Markus; 2000 February
  http://www.pubmedcentral.nih.gov/articlerender.fcgi?artid=86214&rendertype=external

The National Library of Medicine: PubMed

One of the quickest and most comprehensive ways to find academic studies in both English and other languages is to use PubMed, maintained by the National Library of Medicine. The advantage of PubMed over previously

---

[19] The value of PubMed Central, in addition to its role as an archive, lies the availability of data from diverse sources stored in a common format in a single repository. Many journals already have online publishing operations, and there is a growing tendency to publish material online only, to the exclusion of print.

mentioned sources is that it covers a greater number of domestic and foreign references. It is also free to the public.[20] If the publisher has a Web site that offers full text of its journals, PubMed will provide links to that site, as well as to sites offering other related data. User registration, a subscription fee, or some other type of fee may be required to access the full text of articles in some journals.

To generate your own bibliography of studies dealing with Acanthamoeba infection, simply go to the PubMed Web site at **www.ncbi.nlm.nih.gov/pubmed**. Type "Acanthamoeba infection" (or synonyms) into the search box, and click "Go." The following is the type of output you can expect from PubMed for "Acanthamoeba infection" (hyperlinks lead to article summaries):

- **Acanthamoeba infection after radial keratotomy.**
  Author(s): Friedman RF, Wolf TC, Chodosh J.
  Source: American Journal of Ophthalmology. 1997 March; 123(3): 409-10.
  http://www.ncbi.nlm.nih.gov:80/entrez/query.fcgi?cmd=Retrieve&db=PubMed&list_uids=9063258&dopt=Abstract

- **Acanthamoeba infection of peptic ulcer.**
  Author(s): Thamprasert K, Khunamornpong S, Morakote N.
  Source: Annals of Tropical Medicine and Parasitology. 1993 August; 87(4): 403-5. No Abstract Available.
  http://www.ncbi.nlm.nih.gov:80/entrez/query.fcgi?cmd=Retrieve&db=PubMed&list_uids=8250632&dopt=Abstract

- **Acanthamoeba infection presenting as skin lesions in patients with the acquired immunodeficiency syndrome.**
  Author(s): Tan B, Weldon-Linne CM, Rhone DP, Penning CL, Visvesvara GS.
  Source: Archives of Pathology & Laboratory Medicine. 1993 October; 117(10): 1043-6.
  http://www.ncbi.nlm.nih.gov:80/entrez/query.fcgi?cmd=Retrieve&db=PubMed&list_uids=8215828&dopt=Abstract

---

[20] PubMed was developed by the National Center for Biotechnology Information (NCBI) at the National Library of Medicine (NLM) at the National Institutes of Health (NIH). The PubMed database was developed in conjunction with publishers of biomedical literature as a search tool for accessing literature citations and linking to full-text journal articles at Web sites of participating publishers. Publishers that participate in PubMed supply NLM with their citations electronically prior to or at the time of publication.

- **Acanthamoeba infection.**
  Author(s): Wortman PD.
  Source: International Journal of Dermatology. 1996 January; 35(1): 48-51.
  Review. No Abstract Available.
  http://www.ncbi.nlm.nih.gov:80/entrez/query.fcgi?cmd=Retrieve&db=
  PubMed&list_uids=8838931&dopt=Abstract

- **Acquired immunodeficiency syndrome associated with Acanthamoeba infection and other opportunistic organisms.**
  Author(s): Gonzalez MM, Gould E, Dickinson G, Martinez AJ, Visvesvara G, Cleary TJ, Hensley GT.
  Source: Archives of Pathology & Laboratory Medicine. 1986 August; 110(8): 749-51.
  http://www.ncbi.nlm.nih.gov:80/entrez/query.fcgi?cmd=Retrieve&db=
  PubMed&list_uids=3488048&dopt=Abstract

- **Brief report: successful treatment of disseminated acanthamoeba infection in an immunocompromised patient.**
  Author(s): Slater CA, Sickel JZ, Visvesvara GS, Pabico RC, Gaspari AA.
  Source: The New England Journal of Medicine. 1994 July 14; 331(2): 85-7.
  No Abstract Available.
  http://www.ncbi.nlm.nih.gov:80/entrez/query.fcgi?cmd=Retrieve&db=
  PubMed&list_uids=8208270&dopt=Abstract

- **Cutaneous acanthamoeba infection associated with leukocytoclastic vasculitis in an AIDS patient.**
  Author(s): Helton J, Loveless M, White CR Jr.
  Source: The American Journal of Dermatopathology. 1993 April; 15(2): 146-9.
  http://www.ncbi.nlm.nih.gov:80/entrez/query.fcgi?cmd=Retrieve&db=
  PubMed&list_uids=8494115&dopt=Abstract

- **Cutaneous Acanthamoeba infection in the acquired immunodeficiency syndrome: response to multidrug therapy.**
  Author(s): Hunt SJ, Reed SL, Mathews WC, Torian B.
  Source: Cutis. 1995 November; 56(5): 285-7.
  http://www.ncbi.nlm.nih.gov:80/entrez/query.fcgi?cmd=Retrieve&db=
  PubMed&list_uids=8565615&dopt=Abstract

- **Diagnosis of Acanthamoeba infection by cutaneous manifestations in a man seropositive to HIV.**
  Author(s): May LP, Sidhu GS, Buchness MR.

Source: Journal of the American Academy of Dermatology. 1992
February; 26(2 Pt 2): 352-5.
http://www.ncbi.nlm.nih.gov:80/entrez/query.fcgi?cmd=Retrieve&db=
PubMed&list_uids=1569257&dopt=Abstract

- **Disseminated Acanthamoeba infection in a child with symptomatic
  human immunodeficiency virus infection.**
  Author(s): Friedland LR, Raphael SA, Deutsch ES, Johal J, Martyn LJ,
  Visvesvara GS, Lischner HW.
  Source: The Pediatric Infectious Disease Journal. 1992 May; 11(5): 404-7.
  No Abstract Available.
  http://www.ncbi.nlm.nih.gov:80/entrez/query.fcgi?cmd=Retrieve&db=
  PubMed&list_uids=1630862&dopt=Abstract

- **Disseminated acanthamoeba infection in a patient with AIDS:
  response to 5-fluorocytosine therapy.**
  Author(s): Casper T, Basset D, Leclercq C, Fabre J, Peyron-Raison N,
  Reynes J.
  Source: Clinical Infectious Diseases : an Official Publication of the
  Infectious Diseases Society of America. 1999 October; 29(4): 944-5. No
  Abstract Available.
  http://www.ncbi.nlm.nih.gov:80/entrez/query.fcgi?cmd=Retrieve&db=
  PubMed&list_uids=10589923&dopt=Abstract

- **Disseminated acanthamoeba infection in patients with AIDS: case
  reports and review.**
  Author(s): Sison JP, Kemper CA, Loveless M, McShane D, Visvesvara GS,
  Deresinski SC.
  Source: Clinical Infectious Diseases : an Official Publication of the
  Infectious Diseases Society of America. 1995 May; 20(5): 1207-16. Review.
  http://www.ncbi.nlm.nih.gov:80/entrez/query.fcgi?cmd=Retrieve&db=
  PubMed&list_uids=7620001&dopt=Abstract

- **Disseminated granulomatous acanthamoeba infection presenting as an
  unusual skin lesion.**
  Author(s): Gullett J, Mills J, Hadley K, Podemski B, Pitts L, Gelber R.
  Source: The American Journal of Medicine. 1979 November; 67(5): 891-6.
  http://www.ncbi.nlm.nih.gov:80/entrez/query.fcgi?cmd=Retrieve&db=
  PubMed&list_uids=507100&dopt=Abstract

- **Is the intestinal tract a portal of entry for Acanthamoeba infection?**
  Author(s): Sadaka HA, Emam EE.

Source: J Egypt Soc Parasitol. 2001 December; 31(3): 781-90.
http://www.ncbi.nlm.nih.gov:80/entrez/query.fcgi?cmd=Retrieve&db=
PubMed&list_uids=11775104&dopt=Abstract

- **Primary cutaneous acanthamoeba infection in a patient with AIDS.**
  Author(s): Migueles S, Kumar P.
  Source: Clinical Infectious Diseases : an Official Publication of the
  Infectious Diseases Society of America. 1998 December; 27(6): 1547-8. No
  Abstract Available.
  http://www.ncbi.nlm.nih.gov:80/entrez/query.fcgi?cmd=Retrieve&db=
  PubMed&list_uids=9868688&dopt=Abstract

- **The increasing importance of Acanthamoeba infections.**
  Author(s): Marciano-Cabral F, Puffenbarger R, Cabral GA.
  Source: J Eukaryot Microbiol. 2000 January-February; 47(1): 29-36.
  Review.
  http://www.ncbi.nlm.nih.gov:80/entrez/query.fcgi?cmd=Retrieve&db=
  PubMed&list_uids=10651293&dopt=Abstract

- **18S ribosomal DNA typing and tracking of Acanthamoeba species
  isolates from corneal scrape specimens, contact lenses, lens cases, and
  home water supplies of Acanthamoeba keratitis patients in Hong
  Kong.**
  Author(s): Booton GC, Kelly DJ, Chu YW, Seal DV, Houang E, Lam DS,
  Byers TJ, Fuerst PA.
  Source: Journal of Clinical Microbiology. 2002 May; 40(5): 1621-5.
  http://www.ncbi.nlm.nih.gov:80/entrez/query.fcgi?cmd=Retrieve&db=
  PubMed&list_uids=11980931&dopt=Abstract

- **A review of 72 consecutive cases of Acanthamoeba keratitis, 1984-1992.**
  Author(s): Bacon AS, Frazer DG, Dart JK, Matheson M, Ficker LA, Wright
  P.
  Source: Eye (London, England). 1993; 7 (Pt 6): 719-25.
  http://www.ncbi.nlm.nih.gov:80/entrez/query.fcgi?cmd=Retrieve&db=
  PubMed&list_uids=8119418&dopt=Abstract

- **Acanthamoeba keratitis and contact lens wear: the patient is at fault.**
  Author(s): Moore MB.
  Source: Cornea. 1990; 9 Suppl 1: S33-5; Discussion S39-40. Review.
  http://www.ncbi.nlm.nih.gov:80/entrez/query.fcgi?cmd=Retrieve&db=
  PubMed&list_uids=2189677&dopt=Abstract

- **Acanthamoeba keratitis associated with contact lenses; report of three cases in Italy.**
  Author(s): Mancino R, Iori A, Palma S, Corsi A, Cancrini G, Cerulli L.
  Source: Parassitologia. 1997 March; 39(1): 37-40.
  http://www.ncbi.nlm.nih.gov:80/entrez/query.fcgi?cmd=Retrieve&db=PubMed&list_uids=9419845&dopt=Abstract

- **Acanthamoeba keratitis associated with fungal keratitis.**
  Author(s): Froumis NA, Mondino BJ, Glasgow BJ.
  Source: American Journal of Ophthalmology. 2001 April; 131(4): 508-9.
  http://www.ncbi.nlm.nih.gov:80/entrez/query.fcgi?cmd=Retrieve&db=PubMed&list_uids=11292419&dopt=Abstract

- **Acanthamoeba keratitis following optical keratoplasty.**
  Author(s): Panda N, Pushker N, Satpathy G, Naik N.
  Source: Eye (London, England). 1999 August; 13 (Pt 4): 588-9. No Abstract Available.
  http://www.ncbi.nlm.nih.gov:80/entrez/query.fcgi?cmd=Retrieve&db=PubMed&list_uids=10692939&dopt=Abstract

- **Acanthamoeba keratitis in New Zealand, including two cases with in vivo resistance to polyhexamethylene biguanide.**
  Author(s): Murdoch D, Gray TB, Cursons R, Parr D.
  Source: Australian and New Zealand Journal of Ophthalmology. 1998 August; 26(3): 231-6.
  http://www.ncbi.nlm.nih.gov:80/entrez/query.fcgi?cmd=Retrieve&db=PubMed&list_uids=9717755&dopt=Abstract

- **Acanthamoeba keratitis in non-contact lens wearers.**
  Author(s): Sharma S, Srinivasan M, George C.
  Source: Archives of Ophthalmology. 1990 May; 108(5): 676-8.
  http://www.ncbi.nlm.nih.gov:80/entrez/query.fcgi?cmd=Retrieve&db=PubMed&list_uids=2334324&dopt=Abstract

- **Acanthamoeba keratitis in Pondicherry.**
  Author(s): Parija SC, Prakash MR, Rao VA, Vellaniparambil RJ.
  Source: J Commun Dis. 2001 June; 33(2): 126-9.
  http://www.ncbi.nlm.nih.gov:80/entrez/query.fcgi?cmd=Retrieve&db=PubMed&list_uids=12170932&dopt=Abstract

- **Acanthamoeba keratitis in soft contact lens wearers.**
  Author(s): Dornic DI, Wolf T, Dillon WH, Christensen B, Deem CD.

Source: J Am Optom Assoc. 1987 June; 58(6): 482-6.
http://www.ncbi.nlm.nih.gov:80/entrez/query.fcgi?cmd=Retrieve&db=
PubMed&list_uids=3305672&dopt=Abstract

- **Acanthamoeba keratitis in soft contact lens wearers. A case-control study.**
  Author(s): Stehr-Green JK, Bailey TM, Brandt FH, Carr JH, Bond WW, Visvesvara GS.
  Source: Jama : the Journal of the American Medical Association. 1987 July 3; 258(1): 57-60.
  http://www.ncbi.nlm.nih.gov:80/entrez/query.fcgi?cmd=Retrieve&db=
  PubMed&list_uids=3586292&dopt=Abstract

- **Acanthamoeba keratitis in Tennessee: a growing problem in patients wearing contact lenses.**
  Author(s): Johns KJ, Parrish CM, Seal MR, Jerkins GW, Berrie WR, Litchford DW, Sullivan WR, Boone JE, Elliott JH, O'Day DM.
  Source: J Tenn Med Assoc. 1989 November; 82(11): 584-8.
  http://www.ncbi.nlm.nih.gov:80/entrez/query.fcgi?cmd=Retrieve&db=
  PubMed&list_uids=2622154&dopt=Abstract

- **Acanthamoeba keratitis presenting as dendritic keratitis in a soft contact lens wearer.**
  Author(s): Yeung EY, Huang SC, Tsai RJ.
  Source: Chang Gung Med J. 2002 March; 25(3): 201-6.
  http://www.ncbi.nlm.nih.gov:80/entrez/query.fcgi?cmd=Retrieve&db=
  PubMed&list_uids=12022742&dopt=Abstract

- **Acanthamoeba keratitis successfully treated medically.**
  Author(s): Wright P, Warhurst D, Jones BR.
  Source: The British Journal of Ophthalmology. 1985 October; 69(10): 778-82.
  http://www.ncbi.nlm.nih.gov:80/entrez/query.fcgi?cmd=Retrieve&db=
  PubMed&list_uids=4052364&dopt=Abstract

- **Acanthamoeba keratitis successfully treated with penetrating keratoplasty: suggested immunogenic mechanisms of action.**
  Author(s): Blackman HJ, Rao NA, Lemp MA, Visvesvara GS.
  Source: Cornea. 1984; 3(2): 125-30.
  http://www.ncbi.nlm.nih.gov:80/entrez/query.fcgi?cmd=Retrieve&db=
  PubMed&list_uids=6399233&dopt=Abstract

- **Acanthamoeba keratitis with granulomatous reaction involving the stroma and anterior chamber.**
  Author(s): Mietz H, Font RL.
  Source: Archives of Ophthalmology. 1997 February; 115(2): 259-63.
  http://www.ncbi.nlm.nih.gov:80/entrez/query.fcgi?cmd=Retrieve&db=PubMed&list_uids=9046264&dopt=Abstract

- **Acanthamoeba keratitis.**
  Author(s): Illingworth CD, Cook SD.
  Source: Survey of Ophthalmology. 1998 May-June; 42(6): 493-508. Review.
  http://www.ncbi.nlm.nih.gov:80/entrez/query.fcgi?cmd=Retrieve&db=PubMed&list_uids=9635900&dopt=Abstract

- **Acanthamoeba keratitis. A review of the literature.**
  Author(s): Auran JD, Starr MB, Jakobiec FA.
  Source: Cornea. 1987; 6(1): 2-26. Review.
  http://www.ncbi.nlm.nih.gov:80/entrez/query.fcgi?cmd=Retrieve&db=PubMed&list_uids=3556011&dopt=Abstract

- **Acanthamoeba keratitis. Potential role for topical clotrimazole in combination chemotherapy.**
  Author(s): Driebe WT Jr, Stern GA, Epstein RJ, Visvesvara GS, Adi M, Komadina T.
  Source: Archives of Ophthalmology. 1988 September; 106(9): 1196-201.
  http://www.ncbi.nlm.nih.gov:80/entrez/query.fcgi?cmd=Retrieve&db=PubMed&list_uids=3046582&dopt=Abstract

- **Acanthamoeba keratitis. The value of early diagnosis.**
  Author(s): Bacon AS, Dart JK, Ficker LA, Matheson MM, Wright P.
  Source: Ophthalmology. 1993 August; 100(8): 1238-43.
  http://www.ncbi.nlm.nih.gov:80/entrez/query.fcgi?cmd=Retrieve&db=PubMed&list_uids=8341508&dopt=Abstract

- **Acanthamoeba keratitis: a review.**
  Author(s): Claerhout I, Kestelyn P.
  Source: Bull Soc Belge Ophtalmol. 1999; 274: 71-82. Review.
  http://www.ncbi.nlm.nih.gov:80/entrez/query.fcgi?cmd=Retrieve&db=PubMed&list_uids=10670164&dopt=Abstract

- **Acanthamoeba keratitis: a sobering case and a promising new treatment.**
  Author(s): Gray TB, Gross KA, Cursons RT, Shewan JF.
  Source: Australian and New Zealand Journal of Ophthalmology. 1994 February; 22(1): 73-6.
  http://www.ncbi.nlm.nih.gov:80/entrez/query.fcgi?cmd=Retrieve&db= PubMed&list_uids=8037919&dopt=Abstract

- **Acanthamoeba keratitis: first recorded case from a Palestinian patient with trachoma.**
  Author(s): Pyott A, Hay J, Seal D.
  Source: The British Journal of Ophthalmology. 1996 September; 80(9): 849. No Abstract Available.
  http://www.ncbi.nlm.nih.gov:80/entrez/query.fcgi?cmd=Retrieve&db= PubMed&list_uids=8942385&dopt=Abstract

- **Acanthamoeba keratitis: synergy between amebic and bacterial cocontaminants in contact lens care systems as a prelude to infection.**
  Author(s): Bottone EJ, Madayag RM, Qureshi MN.
  Source: Journal of Clinical Microbiology. 1992 September; 30(9): 2447-50.
  http://www.ncbi.nlm.nih.gov:80/entrez/query.fcgi?cmd=Retrieve&db= PubMed&list_uids=1401013&dopt=Abstract

- **Acanthamoeba keratitis--resistance to medical therapy.**
  Author(s): Ficker L, Seal D, Warhurst D, Wright P.
  Source: Eye (London, England). 1990; 4 (Pt 6): 835-8.
  http://www.ncbi.nlm.nih.gov:80/entrez/query.fcgi?cmd=Retrieve&db= PubMed&list_uids=2101116&dopt=Abstract

- **Advances in the management of keratomycosis and Acanthamoeba keratitis.**
  Author(s): O'Day DM, Head WS.
  Source: Cornea. 2000 September; 19(5): 681-7. Review.
  http://www.ncbi.nlm.nih.gov:80/entrez/query.fcgi?cmd=Retrieve&db= PubMed&list_uids=11009320&dopt=Abstract

- **An immortalized hamster corneal epithelial cell line for studies of the pathogenesis of Acanthamoeba keratitis.**
  Author(s): Halenda RM, Grevan VL, Hook RR, Riley LK.

Source: Current Eye Research. 1998 March; 17(3): 225-30.
http://www.ncbi.nlm.nih.gov:80/entrez/query.fcgi?cmd=Retrieve&db=
PubMed&list_uids=9543629&dopt=Abstract

- **Chorioretinitis in the contralateral eye of a patient with Acanthamoeba keratitis.**
  Author(s): Johns KJ, O'Day DM, Feman SS.
  Source: Ophthalmology. 1988 May; 95(5): 635-9.
  http://www.ncbi.nlm.nih.gov:80/entrez/query.fcgi?cmd=Retrieve&db=
  PubMed&list_uids=3050700&dopt=Abstract

- **Clinical signs and medical therapy of early Acanthamoeba keratitis.**
  Author(s): Lindquist TD, Sher NA, Doughman DJ.
  Source: Archives of Ophthalmology. 1988 January; 106(1): 73-7.
  http://www.ncbi.nlm.nih.gov:80/entrez/query.fcgi?cmd=Retrieve&db=
  PubMed&list_uids=3337710&dopt=Abstract

- **Coexistent Acanthamoeba keratitis and herpetic keratitis.**
  Author(s): Mathers WD, Goldberg MA, Sutphin JE, Ditkoff JW, Folberg R.
  Source: Archives of Ophthalmology. 1997 June; 115(6): 714-8.
  http://www.ncbi.nlm.nih.gov:80/entrez/query.fcgi?cmd=Retrieve&db=
  PubMed&list_uids=9194720&dopt=Abstract

- **Coexistent adenoviral keratoconjunctivitis and Acanthamoeba keratitis.**
  Author(s): Gajdatsy AD, Kosmin A, Barrett GD.
  Source: Clinical & Experimental Ophthalmology. 2000 December; 28(6): 434-6.
  http://www.ncbi.nlm.nih.gov:80/entrez/query.fcgi?cmd=Retrieve&db=
  PubMed&list_uids=11202467&dopt=Abstract

- **Confocal microscopy findings of Acanthamoeba keratitis.**
  Author(s): Pfister DR, Cameron JD, Krachmer JH, Holland EJ.
  Source: American Journal of Ophthalmology. 1996 February; 121(2): 119-28.
  http://www.ncbi.nlm.nih.gov:80/entrez/query.fcgi?cmd=Retrieve&db=
  PubMed&list_uids=8623881&dopt=Abstract

- **Elevated corneal epithelial lines in Acanthamoeba keratitis.**
  Author(s): Florakis GJ, Folberg R, Krachmer JH, Tse DT, Roussel TJ, Vrabec MP.

Source: Archives of Ophthalmology. 1988 September; 106(9): 1202-6.
http://www.ncbi.nlm.nih.gov:80/entrez/query.fcgi?cmd=Retrieve&db=
PubMed&list_uids=3046583&dopt=Abstract

- **Exacerbation of Acanthamoeba keratitis in animals treated with anti-macrophage inflammatory protein 2 or antineutrophil antibodies.**
  Author(s): Hurt M, Apte S, Leher H, Howard K, Niederkorn J, Alizadeh H.
  Source: Infection and Immunity. 2001 May; 69(5): 2988-95.
  http://www.ncbi.nlm.nih.gov:80/entrez/query.fcgi?cmd=Retrieve&db=
  PubMed&list_uids=11292716&dopt=Abstract

- **Exfoliated cytopathology of Acanthamoeba keratitis.**
  Author(s): Margo CE, Brinser JH, Groden L.
  Source: Jama : the Journal of the American Medical Association. 1986 April 25; 255(16): 2216. No Abstract Available.
  http://www.ncbi.nlm.nih.gov:80/entrez/query.fcgi?cmd=Retrieve&db=
  PubMed&list_uids=3959306&dopt=Abstract

- **Experimental Acanthamoeba keratitis: I. Preliminary findings.**
  Author(s): Larkin DF, Easty DL.
  Source: The British Journal of Ophthalmology. 1990 September; 74(9): 551-5.
  http://www.ncbi.nlm.nih.gov:80/entrez/query.fcgi?cmd=Retrieve&db=
  PubMed&list_uids=2393646&dopt=Abstract

- **Immunopathology and electron microscopy of Acanthamoeba keratitis.**
  Author(s): Mathers W, Stevens G Jr, Rodrigues M, Chan CC, Gold J, Visvesvara GS, Lemp MA, Zimmerman LE.
  Source: American Journal of Ophthalmology. 1987 May 15; 103(5): 626-35.
  http://www.ncbi.nlm.nih.gov:80/entrez/query.fcgi?cmd=Retrieve&db=
  PubMed&list_uids=3555096&dopt=Abstract

- **Laboratory diagnosis of Acanthamoeba keratitis using buffered charcoal-yeast extract agar.**
  Author(s): Penland RL, Wilhelmus KR.
  Source: American Journal of Ophthalmology. 1998 October; 126(4): 590-2.
  http://www.ncbi.nlm.nih.gov:80/entrez/query.fcgi?cmd=Retrieve&db=
  PubMed&list_uids=9780107&dopt=Abstract

- **Laboratory investigation of Acanthamoeba keratitis.**
  Author(s): Kilvington S, Larkin DF, White DG, Beeching JR.

Source: Journal of Clinical Microbiology. 1990 December; 28(12): 2722-5.
http://www.ncbi.nlm.nih.gov:80/entrez/query.fcgi?cmd=Retrieve&db=
PubMed&list_uids=1980681&dopt=Abstract

- **Management of Acanthamoeba keratitis. A case report and review of the literature.**
Author(s): Hirst LW, Green WR, Merz W, Kaufmann C, Visvesvara GS, Jensen A, Howard M.
Source: Ophthalmology. 1984 September; 91(9): 1105-11.
http://www.ncbi.nlm.nih.gov:80/entrez/query.fcgi?cmd=Retrieve&db=
PubMed&list_uids=6093021&dopt=Abstract

- **Management of contact lens associated Acanthamoeba keratitis.**
Author(s): Doren GS, Cohen EJ, Higgins SE, Udell IJ, Eagle RC Jr, Arentsen JJ, Laibson PR.
Source: The Clao Journal : Official Publication of the Contact Lens Association of Ophthalmologists, Inc. 1991 April; 17(2): 120-5.
http://www.ncbi.nlm.nih.gov:80/entrez/query.fcgi?cmd=Retrieve&db=
PubMed&list_uids=2049820&dopt=Abstract

- **Management of herpes simplex keratitis: problems associated with epithelial disease.**
Author(s): O'Day DM.
Source: Australian and New Zealand Journal of Ophthalmology. 1987 November; 15(4): 263-7.
http://www.ncbi.nlm.nih.gov:80/entrez/query.fcgi?cmd=Retrieve&db=
PubMed&list_uids=3435669&dopt=Abstract

- **Medical and surgical treatment of Acanthamoeba keratitis.**
Author(s): Cohen EJ, Parlato CJ, Arentsen JJ, Genvert GI, Eagle RC Jr, Wieland MR, Laibson PR.
Source: American Journal of Ophthalmology. 1987 May 15; 103(5): 615-25.
http://www.ncbi.nlm.nih.gov:80/entrez/query.fcgi?cmd=Retrieve&db=
PubMed&list_uids=3555095&dopt=Abstract

- **Monoclonal IgA antibodies protect against Acanthamoeba keratitis.**
Author(s): Leher H, Zaragoza F, Taherzadeh S, Alizadeh H, Niederkorn JY.
Source: Experimental Eye Research. 1999 July; 69(1): 75-84.
http://www.ncbi.nlm.nih.gov:80/entrez/query.fcgi?cmd=Retrieve&db=
PubMed&list_uids=10375451&dopt=Abstract

- **Nonulcerating bacterial keratitis associated with soft and rigid contact lens wear.**
  Author(s): McLeod SD, Goei SL, Taglia DP, McMahon TT.
  Source: Ophthalmology. 1998 March; 105(3): 517-21.
  http://www.ncbi.nlm.nih.gov:80/entrez/query.fcgi?cmd=Retrieve&db=PubMed&list_uids=9499784&dopt=Abstract

- **Oral itraconazole and topical miconazole with debridement for Acanthamoeba keratitis.**
  Author(s): Ishibashi Y, Matsumoto Y, Kabata T, Watanabe R, Hommura S, Yasuraoka K, Ishii K.
  Source: American Journal of Ophthalmology. 1990 February 15; 109(2): 121-6.
  http://www.ncbi.nlm.nih.gov:80/entrez/query.fcgi?cmd=Retrieve&db=PubMed&list_uids=2154105&dopt=Abstract

- **Pathogenesis of Acanthamoeba keratitis: carbohydrate-mediated host-parasite interactions.**
  Author(s): Yang Z, Cao Z, Panjwani N.
  Source: Infection and Immunity. 1997 February; 65(2): 439-45.
  http://www.ncbi.nlm.nih.gov:80/entrez/query.fcgi?cmd=Retrieve&db=PubMed&list_uids=9009294&dopt=Abstract

- **Persistence of acanthamoeba antigen following acanthamoeba keratitis.**
  Author(s): Yang YF, Matheson M, Dart JK, Cree IA.
  Source: The British Journal of Ophthalmology. 2001 March; 85(3): 277-80.
  http://www.ncbi.nlm.nih.gov:80/entrez/query.fcgi?cmd=Retrieve&db=PubMed&list_uids=11222330&dopt=Abstract

- **Polymerase chain reaction analysis of corneal epithelial and tear samples in the diagnosis of Acanthamoeba keratitis.**
  Author(s): Lehmann OJ, Green SM, Morlet N, Kilvington S, Keys MF, Matheson MM, Dart JK, McGill JI, Watt PJ.
  Source: Investigative Ophthalmology & Visual Science. 1998 June; 39(7): 1261-5.
  http://www.ncbi.nlm.nih.gov:80/entrez/query.fcgi?cmd=Retrieve&db=PubMed&list_uids=9620088&dopt=Abstract

- **Polymerase chain reaction diagnosis in fungal keratitis caused by Alternaria alternata.**
  Author(s): Ferrer C, Munoz G, Alio JL, Abad JL, Colomm F.

Source: American Journal of Ophthalmology. 2002 March; 133(3): 398-9.
http://www.ncbi.nlm.nih.gov:80/entrez/query.fcgi?cmd=Retrieve&db=
PubMed&list_uids=11860977&dopt=Abstract

- **Prognosis for keratoplasty in Acanthamoeba keratitis.**
  Author(s): Ficker LA, Kirkness C, Wright P.
  Source: Ophthalmology. 1993 January; 100(1): 105-10.
  http://www.ncbi.nlm.nih.gov:80/entrez/query.fcgi?cmd=Retrieve&db=
  PubMed&list_uids=8433814&dopt=Abstract

- **Recent advances in the treatment of Acanthamoeba keratitis.**
  Author(s): Kumar R, Lloyd D.
  Source: Clinical Infectious Diseases : an Official Publication of the
  Infectious Diseases Society of America. 2002 August 15; 35(4): 434-41.
  Review.
  http://www.ncbi.nlm.nih.gov:80/entrez/query.fcgi?cmd=Retrieve&db=
  PubMed&list_uids=12145728&dopt=Abstract

- **Results of a trial of combined propamidine isethionate and neomycin
  therapy for Acanthamoeba keratitis. Brolene Study Group.**
  Author(s): Hargrave SL, McCulley JP, Husseini Z.
  Source: Ophthalmology. 1999 May; 106(5): 952-7.
  http://www.ncbi.nlm.nih.gov:80/entrez/query.fcgi?cmd=Retrieve&db=
  PubMed&list_uids=10328395&dopt=Abstract

- **Role of mucosal IgA in the resistance to Acanthamoeba keratitis.**
  Author(s): Leher HF, Alizadeh H, Taylor WM, Shea AS, Silvany RS, Van
  Klink F, Jager MJ, Niederkorn JY.
  Source: Investigative Ophthalmology & Visual Science. 1998 December;
  39(13): 2666-73.
  http://www.ncbi.nlm.nih.gov:80/entrez/query.fcgi?cmd=Retrieve&db=
  PubMed&list_uids=9856776&dopt=Abstract

- **Spontaneous corneal graft ulcerative perforation due to mixed
  Acanthamoeba and herpes simplex keratitis: a clinicopathologic study.**
  Author(s): Rumelt S, Cohen I, Rehany U.
  Source: Cornea. 2000 March; 19(2): 240-2. No Abstract Available.
  http://www.ncbi.nlm.nih.gov:80/entrez/query.fcgi?cmd=Retrieve&db=
  PubMed&list_uids=10746460&dopt=Abstract

- **Subepithelial infiltrates in Acanthamoeba keratitis.**
  Author(s): Holland EJ, Alul IH, Meisler DM, Epstein RJ, Rotkis WM, Nathenson AL, Liesegang TJ.
  Source: American Journal of Ophthalmology. 1991 October 15; 112(4): 414-8.
  http://www.ncbi.nlm.nih.gov:80/entrez/query.fcgi?cmd=Retrieve&db=PubMed&list_uids=1928244&dopt=Abstract

- **Successful immunization against Acanthamoeba keratitis in a pig model.**
  Author(s): Alizadeh H, He Y, McCulley JP, Ma D, Stewart GL, Via M, Haehling E, Niederkorn JY.
  Source: Cornea. 1995 March; 14(2): 180-6.
  http://www.ncbi.nlm.nih.gov:80/entrez/query.fcgi?cmd=Retrieve&db=PubMed&list_uids=7743802&dopt=Abstract

- **Successful medical management of Acanthamoeba keratitis.**
  Author(s): Berger ST, Mondino BJ, Hoft RH, Donzis PB, Holland GN, Farley MK, Levenson JE.
  Source: American Journal of Ophthalmology. 1990 October 15; 110(4): 395-403.
  http://www.ncbi.nlm.nih.gov:80/entrez/query.fcgi?cmd=Retrieve&db=PubMed&list_uids=2220974&dopt=Abstract

- **Successful medical therapy of Acanthamoeba keratitis with topical chlorhexidine and propamidine.**
  Author(s): Seal D, Hay J, Kirkness C, Morrell A, Booth A, Tullo A, Ridgway A, Armstrong M.
  Source: Eye (London, England). 1996; 10 (Pt 4): 413-21.
  http://www.ncbi.nlm.nih.gov:80/entrez/query.fcgi?cmd=Retrieve&db=PubMed&list_uids=8944089&dopt=Abstract

- **Successful medical treatment of Acanthamoeba keratitis.**
  Author(s): Azuara-Blanco A, Sadiq AS, Hussain M, Lloyd JH, Dua HS.
  Source: International Ophthalmology. 1997-98; 21(4): 223-7.
  http://www.ncbi.nlm.nih.gov:80/entrez/query.fcgi?cmd=Retrieve&db=PubMed&list_uids=9700010&dopt=Abstract

- **Systemic immune response to Acanthamoeba keratitis in the Chinese hamster.**
  Author(s): Van Klink F, Leher H, Jager MJ, Alizadeh H, Taylor W, Niederkorn JY.

Source: Ocular Immunology and Inflammation. 1997 December; 5(4): 235-44.

http://www.ncbi.nlm.nih.gov:80/entrez/query.fcgi?cmd=Retrieve&db=PubMed&list_uids=9455740&dopt=Abstract

- **The diagnosis and management of Acanthamoeba keratitis.**
  Author(s): McCulley JP, Alizadeh H, Niederkorn JY.
  Source: The Clao Journal : Official Publication of the Contact Lens Association of Ophthalmologists, Inc. 2000 January; 26(1): 47-51. Review.
  http://www.ncbi.nlm.nih.gov:80/entrez/query.fcgi?cmd=Retrieve&db=PubMed&list_uids=10656311&dopt=Abstract

- **The epidemic of Acanthamoeba keratitis: where do we stand?**
  Author(s): Schaumberg DA, Snow KK, Dana MR.
  Source: Cornea. 1998 January; 17(1): 3-10. Review.
  http://www.ncbi.nlm.nih.gov:80/entrez/query.fcgi?cmd=Retrieve&db=PubMed&list_uids=9436873&dopt=Abstract

- **The pathogenesis of Acanthamoeba keratitis.**
  Author(s): Niederkorn JY, Alizadeh H, Leher H, McCulley JP.
  Source: Microbes and Infection / Institut Pasteur. 1999 May; 1(6): 437-43. Review.
  http://www.ncbi.nlm.nih.gov:80/entrez/query.fcgi?cmd=Retrieve&db=PubMed&list_uids=10602676&dopt=Abstract

- **The role of contact lenses, trauma, and Langerhans cells in a Chinese hamster model of Acanthamoeba keratitis.**
  Author(s): van Klink F, Alizadeh H, He Y, Mellon JA, Silvany RE, McCulley JP, Niederkorn JY.
  Source: Investigative Ophthalmology & Visual Science. 1993 May; 34(6): 1937-44.
  http://www.ncbi.nlm.nih.gov:80/entrez/query.fcgi?cmd=Retrieve&db=PubMed&list_uids=8491547&dopt=Abstract

- **The role of macrophages in Acanthamoeba keratitis.**
  Author(s): van Klink F, Taylor WM, Alizadeh H, Jager MJ, van Rooijen N, Niederkorn JY.
  Source: Investigative Ophthalmology & Visual Science. 1996 June; 37(7): 1271-81.
  http://www.ncbi.nlm.nih.gov:80/entrez/query.fcgi?cmd=Retrieve&db=PubMed&list_uids=8641830&dopt=Abstract

- **The role of steroids in the management of Acanthamoeba keratitis, fungal keratitis, and epidemic keratoconjunctivitis.**
  Author(s): Pineda R 2nd, Dohlman CH.
  Source: International Ophthalmology Clinics. 1994 Summer; 34(3): 19-31. Review. No Abstract Available.
  http://www.ncbi.nlm.nih.gov:80/entrez/query.fcgi?cmd=Retrieve&db=PubMed&list_uids=7960514&dopt=Abstract

- **The role of the innate and adaptive immune responses in Acanthamoeba keratitis.**
  Author(s): Niederkorn JY.
  Source: Arch Immunol Ther Exp (Warsz). 2002; 50(1): 53-9. Review.
  http://www.ncbi.nlm.nih.gov:80/entrez/query.fcgi?cmd=Retrieve&db=PubMed&list_uids=11916309&dopt=Abstract

- **The role of topical corticosteroids in the management of Acanthamoeba keratitis.**
  Author(s): Park DH, Palay DA, Daya SM, Stulting RD, Krachmer JH, Holland EJ.
  Source: Cornea. 1997 May; 16(3): 277-83.
  http://www.ncbi.nlm.nih.gov:80/entrez/query.fcgi?cmd=Retrieve&db=PubMed&list_uids=9143798&dopt=Abstract

- **Treatment of Acanthamoeba keratitis combined with fungal infection with polyhexamethylene biguanide.**
  Author(s): Tien SH, Sheu MM.
  Source: Kaohsiung J Med Sci. 1999 November; 15(11): 665-73.
  http://www.ncbi.nlm.nih.gov:80/entrez/query.fcgi?cmd=Retrieve&db=PubMed&list_uids=10630064&dopt=Abstract

- **Treatment of Acanthamoeba keratitis with polyhexamethylene biguanide.**
  Author(s): Larkin DF, Kilvington S, Dart JK.
  Source: Ophthalmology. 1992 February; 99(2): 185-91.
  http://www.ncbi.nlm.nih.gov:80/entrez/query.fcgi?cmd=Retrieve&db=PubMed&list_uids=1553206&dopt=Abstract

- **Treatment of advanced acanthamoeba keratitis with deep lamellar keratectomy and conjunctival flap.**
  Author(s): Cremona G, Carrasco MA, Tytiun A, Cosentino MJ.

Vocabulary Builder

Acyclovir: Functional analog of the nucleoside guanosine. It acts as an antimetabolite, especially in viruses. It is used as an antiviral agent, especially in herpes infections. [NIH]

Antigen: Any substance which is capable, under appropriate conditions, of inducing a specific immune response and of reacting with the products of that response, that is, with specific antibody or specifically sensitized T-lymphocytes, or both. Antigens may be soluble substances, such as toxins and foreign proteins, or particulate, such as bacteria and tissue cells; however, only the portion of the protein or polysaccharide molecule known as the antigenic determinant (q.v.) combines with antibody or a specific receptor on a lymphocyte. Abbreviated Ag. [EU]

Antiviral: Destroying viruses or suppressing their replication. [EU]

Arteries: The vessels carrying blood away from the heart. [NIH]

Assay: Determination of the amount of a particular constituent of a mixture, or of the biological or pharmacological potency of a drug. [EU]

Cannabinoids: Compounds extracted from Cannabis sativa L. and metabolites having the cannabinoid structure. The most active constituents are tetrahydrocannabinol, cannabinol, and cannabidiol. [NIH]

Chemotaxis: The movement of cells or organisms toward or away from a substance in response to its concentration gradient. [NIH]

Chimera: An individual that contains cell populations derived from different zygotes. [NIH]

Cryptosporidium: A genus of coccidian parasites of the family cryptosporidiidae, found in the intestinal epithelium of many vertebrates including humans. [NIH]

Cytokines: Non-antibody proteins secreted by inflammatory leukocytes and some non-leukocytic cells, that act as intercellular mediators. They differ from classical hormones in that they are produced by a number of tissue or cell types rather than by specialized glands. They generally act locally in a paracrine or autocrine rather than endocrine manner. [NIH]

Cytomegalovirus: A genus of the family herpesviridae, subfamily betaherpesvirinae, infecting the salivary glands, liver, spleen, lungs, eyes, and other organs, in which they produce characteristically enlarged cells with intranuclear inclusions. Infection with Cytomegalovirus is also seen as an opportunistic infection in AIDS. [NIH]

Dementia: An acquired organic mental disorder with loss of intellectual abilities of sufficient severity to interfere with social or occupational functioning. The dysfunction is multifaceted and involves memory, behavior, personality, judgment, attention, spatial relations, language, abstract thought, and other executive functions. The intellectual decline is usually progressive, and initially spares the level of consciousness. [NIH]

Electrophysiological: Pertaining to electrophysiology, that is a branch of physiology that is concerned with the electric phenomena associated with living bodies and involved in their functional activity. [EU]

Embryo: In animals, those derivatives of the fertilized ovum that eventually become the offspring, during their period of most rapid development, i.e., after the long axis appears until all major structures are represented. In man, the developing organism is an embryo from about two weeks after fertilization to the end of seventh or eighth week. [EU]

Epitopes: Sites on an antigen that interact with specific antibodies. [NIH]

Exogenous: Developed or originating outside the organism, as exogenous disease. [EU]

Extracellular: Outside a cell or cells. [EU]

Ganglia: Clusters of multipolar neurons surrounded by a capsule of loosely organized connective tissue located outside the central nervous system. [NIH]

Genotype: The genetic constitution of the individual; the characterization of the genes. [NIH]

Helicobacter: A genus of gram-negative, spiral-shaped bacteria that is pathogenic and has been isolated from the intestinal tract of mammals, including humans. [NIH]

Hepatitis: Inflammation of the liver. [EU]

Homologous: Corresponding in structure, position, origin, etc., as (a) the feathers of a bird and the scales of a fish, (b) antigen and its specific antibody, (c) allelic chromosomes. [EU]

Hybridization: The genetic process of crossbreeding to produce a hybrid. Hybrid nucleic acids can be formed by nucleic acid hybridization of DNA and RNA molecules. Protein hybridization allows for hybrid proteins to be formed from polypeptide chains. [NIH]

Hygienic: Pertaining to hygiene, or conducive to health. [EU]

Immunity: The condition of being immune; the protection against infectious disease conferred either by the immune response generated by immunization or previous infection or by other nonimmunologic factors (innate i.). [EU]

Immunohistochemistry: Histochemical localization of immunoreactive substances using labeled antibodies as reagents. [NIH]

Infiltration: The diffusion or accumulation in a tissue or cells of substances not normal to it or in amounts of the normal. Also, the material so accumulated. [EU]

Inflammation: A pathological process characterized by injury or destruction of tissues caused by a variety of cytologic and chemical reactions. It is usually manifested by typical signs of pain, heat, redness, swelling, and loss of function. [NIH]

Interneurons: Most generally any neurons which are not motor or sensory. Interneurons may also refer to neurons whose axons remain within a particular brain region as contrasted with projection neurons which have axons projecting to other brain regions. [NIH]

Kinetic: Pertaining to or producing motion. [EU]

Lobe: A more or less well-defined portion of any organ, especially of the brain, lungs, and glands. Lobes are demarcated by fissures, sulci, connective tissue, and by their shape. [EU]

Lymphocytic: Pertaining to, characterized by, or of the nature of lymphocytes. [EU]

Molecular: Of, pertaining to, or composed of molecules : a very small mass of matter. [EU]

Mononucleosis: The presence of an abnormally large number of mononuclear leucocytes (monocytes) in the blood. The term is often used alone to refer to infectious mononucleosis. [EU]

Neurology: A medical specialty concerned with the study of the structures, functions, and diseases of the nervous system. [NIH]

Neutrophil: Having an affinity for neutral dyes. [EU]

Ocular: 1. of, pertaining to, or affecting the eye. 2. eyepiece. [EU]

Osmolarity: The concentration of osmotically active particles expressed in terms of osmoles of solute per litre of solution. [EU]

Parenchyma: The essential elements of an organ; used in anatomical nomenclature as a general term to designate the functional elements of an organ, as distinguished from its framework, or stroma. [EU]

Parvovirus: A genus of the family parvoviridae, subfamily parvovirinae, infecting a variety of vertebrates including humans. Parvoviruses are responsible for a number of important diseases but also can be nonpathogenic in certain hosts. The type species is mice minute virus. [NIH]

Pathogen: Any disease-producing microorganism. [EU]

Perinatal: Pertaining to or occurring in the period shortly before and after birth; variously defined as beginning with completion of the twentieth to twenty-eighth week of gestation and ending 7 to 28 days after birth. [EU]

Phagocytosis: Endocytosis of particulate material, such as microorganisms or cell fragments. The material is taken into the cell in membrane-bound vesicles (phagosomes) that originate as pinched off invaginations of the plasma membrane. Phagosomes fuse with lysosomes, forming phagolysosomes in which the engulfed material is killed and digested. [EU]

Pharyngitis: Inflammation of the pharynx. [EU]

Phenotype: The outward appearance of the individual. It is the product of interactions between genes and between the genotype and the environment. This includes the killer phenotype, characteristic of yeasts. [NIH]

Placenta: A highly vascular fetal organ through which the fetus absorbs oxygen and other nutrients and excretes carbon dioxide and other wastes. It begins to form about the eighth day of gestation when the blastocyst adheres to the decidua. [NIH]

Pneumonia: Inflammation of the lungs with consolidation. [EU]

Postnatal: Occurring after birth, with reference to the newborn. [EU]

Prenatal: Existing or occurring before birth, with reference to the fetus. [EU]

Prevalence: The total number of cases of a given disease in a specified population at a designated time. It is differentiated from incidence, which refers to the number of new cases in the population at a given time. [NIH]

Prophylaxis: The prevention of disease; preventive treatment. [EU]

Proteins: Polymers of amino acids linked by peptide bonds. The specific sequence of amino acids determines the shape and function of the protein. [NIH]

Pseudomonas: A genus of gram-negative, aerobic, rod-shaped bacteria widely distributed in nature. Some species are pathogenic for humans, animals, and plants. [NIH]

Psychiatry: The medical science that deals with the origin, diagnosis, prevention, and treatment of mental disorders. [NIH]

Pulmonary: Pertaining to the lungs. [EU]

Receptor: 1. a molecular structure within a cell or on the surface characterized by (1) selective binding of a specific substance and (2) a specific physiologic effect that accompanies the binding, e.g., cell-surface receptors for peptide hormones, neurotransmitters, antigens, complement fragments, and immunoglobulins and cytoplasmic receptors for steroid hormones. 2. a sensory nerve terminal that responds to stimuli of various kinds. [EU]

Recombinant: 1. a cell or an individual with a new combination of genes not found together in either parent; usually applied to linked genes. [EU]

Sarcoma: A tumour made up of a substance like the embryonic connective tissue; tissue composed of closely packed cells embedded in a fibrillar or homogeneous substance. Sarcomas are often highly malignant. [EU]

Schizophrenia: A severe emotional disorder of psychotic depth characteristically marked by a retreat from reality with delusion formation, hallucinations, emotional disharmony, and regressive behavior. [NIH]

Sclerosis: A induration, or hardening; especially hardening of a part from inflammation and in diseases of the interstitial substance. The term is used chiefly for such a hardening of the nervous system due to hyperplasia of the connective tissue or to designate hardening of the blood vessels. [EU]

Seroconversion: The change of a serologic test from negative to positive, indicating the development of antibodies in response to infection or immunization. [EU]

Serology: The study of serum, especially of antigen-antibody reactions in vitro. [NIH]

Spermicide: An agent that is destructive to spermatozoa. [EU]

Spores: The reproductive elements of lower organisms, such as protozoa, fungi, and cryptogamic plants. [NIH]

Subarachnoid: Situated or occurring between the arachnoid and the pia mater. [EU]

Subclinical: Without clinical manifestations; said of the early stage(s) of an infection or other disease or abnormality before symptoms and signs become apparent or detectable by clinical examination or laboratory tests, or of a very mild form of an infection or other disease or abnormality. [EU]

Sulfadiazine: A short-acting sulfonamide used in combination with pyrimethamine to treat toxoplasmosis in patients with acquired immunodeficiency syndrome and in newborns with congenital infections. [NIH]

Superinfection: A new infection complicating the course of antimicrobial therapy of an existing infectious process, and resulting from invasion by bacteria or fungi resistant to the drug(s) in use. It may occur at the site of the original infection or at a remote site. [EU]

Symptomatic: 1. pertaining to or of the nature of a symptom. 2. indicative (of a particular disease or disorder). 3. exhibiting the symptoms of a particular disease but having a different cause. 4. directed at the allying of symptoms, as symptomatic treatment. [EU]

Tolerance: 1. the ability to endure unusually large doses of a drug or toxin. 2. acquired drug tolerance; a decreasing response to repeated constant doses of a drug or the need for increasing doses to maintain a constant response. [EU]

Toxicology: The science concerned with the detection, chemical composition, and pharmacologic action of toxic substances or poisons and the treatment and prevention of toxic manifestations. [NIH]

Vaccine: A suspension of attenuated or killed microorganisms (bacteria, viruses, or rickettsiae), administered for the prevention, amelioration or treatment of infectious diseases. [EU]

Vaginal: 1. of the nature of a sheath; ensheathing. 2. pertaining to the vagina. 3. pertaining to the tunica vaginalis testis. [EU]

Ventricular: Pertaining to a ventricle. [EU]

Viral: Pertaining to, caused by, or of the nature of virus. [EU]

Viremia: The presence of viruses in the blood. [NIH]

Virion: The infective system of a virus, composed of the viral genome, a protein core, and a protein coat called a capsid, which may be naked or enclosed in a lipoprotein envelope called the peplos. [NIH]

CHAPTER 4. BOOKS ON ACANTHAMOEBA INFECTION

Overview

This chapter provides bibliographic book references relating to Acanthamoeba infection. You have many options to locate books on Acanthamoeba infection. The simplest method is to go to your local bookseller and inquire about titles that they have in stock or can special order for you. Some patients, however, feel uncomfortable approaching their local booksellers and prefer online sources (e.g. **www.amazon.com** and **www.bn.com**). In addition to online booksellers, excellent sources for book titles on Acanthamoeba infection include the Combined Health Information Database and the National Library of Medicine. Once you have found a title that interests you, visit your local public or medical library to see if it is available for loan.

The National Library of Medicine Book Index

The National Library of Medicine at the National Institutes of Health has a massive database of books published on healthcare and biomedicine. Go to the following Internet site, **http://locatorplus.gov/**, and then select "Search LOCATORplus." Once you are in the search area, simply type "Acanthamoeba infection" (or synonyms) into the search box, and select "books only." From there, results can be sorted by publication date, author, or relevance. The following was recently catalogued by the National Library of Medicine:[21]

- **Communicable diseases: policy and procedure, implementation, and education.** Author: Marguerite A. Bouvette; Year: 1998; Bossier City, LA: Professional Printing & Publishing, Inc., c1998; ISBN: 0929442342
  http://www.amazon.com/exec/obidos/ASIN/0929442342/icongroupin terna

- **Firepower in the lab: automation in the fight against infectious diseases and bioterrorism.** Author: Scott P. Layne, Tony J. Beugelsdijk, and D. Kumar N. Patel, editors; Year: 2001; Washington D.C.: Joseph Henry Press, c2001; ISBN: 0309068495
  http://www.amazon.com/exec/obidos/ASIN/0309068495/icongroupin terna

- **Guide to infection control in the hospital.** Author: R. Wenzel ... [et al.]; Year: 1998; Hamilton, Ont.: B.C. Decker; Malden, MA: Blackwell Science [U.S. distributor], 1998; ISBN: 1550090593
  http://www.amazon.com/exec/obidos/ASIN/1550090593/icongroupin terna

- **Infection control in clinical practice.** Author: Jennie Wilson; foreword by Liz A. Jenner; Year: 2001; New York: Bailliere Tindall, 2001; ISBN: 0702025542
  http://www.amazon.com/exec/obidos/ASIN/0702025542/icongroupin terna

- **Infection highlights, 2000-01.** Author: edited by Mark H. Wilcox; Year: 2001; Oxford: Health Press, c2001; ISBN: 1899541942
  http://www.amazon.com/exec/obidos/ASIN/1899541942/icongroupin terna

- **Infection in the critically ill: an ongoing challenge.** Author: Van Saene, H.K.F., Sganga, G., Silvestri, L., eds; Year: 2001; Milano; New York: Springer, c2001; ISBN: 8847001382 (pbk.)
  http://www.amazon.com/exec/obidos/ASIN/8847001382/icongroupin terna

---

[21] In addition to LOCATORPlus, in collaboration with authors and publishers, the National Center for Biotechnology Information (NCBI) is adapting biomedical books for the Web. The books may be accessed in two ways: (1) by searching directly using any search term or phrase (in the same way as the bibliographic database PubMed), or (2) by following the links to PubMed abstracts. Each PubMed abstract has a "Books" button that displays a facsimile of the abstract in which some phrases are hypertext links. These phrases are also found in the books available at NCBI. Click on hyperlinked results in the list of books in which the phrase is found. Currently, the majority of the links are between the books and PubMed. In the future, more links will be created between the books and other types of information, such as gene and protein sequences and macromolecular structures. See **http://www.ncbi.nlm.nih.gov/entrez/query.fcgi?db=Books.**

- **Infection prevention in surgical settings.** Author: Barbara J. Gruendemann, Sandra Stonehocker Mangum; Year: 2001; Philadelphia: W.B. Saunders Co., c2001; ISBN: 0721690351
  http://www.amazon.com/exec/obidos/ASIN/0721690351/icongroupin terna

- **Managing difficult infections.** Author: edited by R. C. Read; Year: 1999; London: Science Press, c1999; ISBN: 1858733146

Chapters on Acanthamoeba Infection

Frequently, Acanthamoeba infection will be discussed within a book, perhaps within a specific chapter. In order to find chapters that are specifically dealing with Acanthamoeba infection, an excellent source of abstracts is the Combined Health Information Database. You will need to limit your search to book chapters and Acanthamoeba infection using the "Detailed Search" option. Go directly to the following hyperlink: **http://chid.nih.gov/detail/detail.html**. To find book chapters, use the drop boxes at the bottom of the search page where "You may refine your search by." Select the dates and language you prefer, and the format option "Book Chapter." By making these selections and typing in "Acanthamoeba infection" (or synonyms) into the "For these words:" box, you will only receive results on chapters in books.

General Home References

In addition to references for Acanthamoeba infection, you may want a general home medical guide that spans all aspects of home healthcare. The following list is a recent sample of such guides (sorted alphabetically by title; hyperlinks provide rankings, information, and reviews at Amazon.com):

- **Encyclopedia of Infectious Diseases (Encyclopedia of Infectious Diseases, 1998)** by Carol Turkington, Bonnie Ashby; Library Binding - 384 pages (September 1998), Facts on File, Inc.; ISBN: 0816035121;
  http://www.amazon.com/exec/obidos/ASIN/0816035121/icongroupinterna

- **Epidemic! The World of Infectious Disease** by Rob Desalle (Editor), American Museum of Natural History; Paperback - 246 pages, 1st edition (September 1999), New Press; ISBN: 1565845463;
  http://www.amazon.com/exec/obidos/ASIN/1565845463/icongroupinterna

- **Outbreak Alert: Responding to the Increasing Threat of Infectious Diseases** by Jason Eberhart-Phillips, M.D.; Paperback - 292 pages (July 2000), New Harbinger Publications; ISBN: 1572242019; http://www.amazon.com/exec/obidos/ASIN/1572242019/icongroupinterna

- **Plague Time: How Stealth Infections Are Causing Cancers, Heart Disease, and Other Deadly Ailments** by Paul W. Ewald; Hardcover - 288 pages (November 2000), Free Press; ISBN: 0684869004; http://www.amazon.com/exec/obidos/ASIN/0684869004/icongroupinterna

Vocabulary Builder

Bioterrorism: The use of biological agents in terrorism. This includes the malevolent use of bacteria, viruses, or toxins against people, animals, or plants. [NIH]

Immunotherapy: Manipulation of the host's immune system in treatment of disease. It includes both active and passive immunization as well as immunosuppressive therapy to prevent graft rejection. [NIH]

Mycobacterium: An organism of the genus Mycobacterium. [EU]

Neonatal: Pertaining to the first four weeks after birth. [EU]

Orthopaedic: Pertaining to the correction of deformities of the musculoskeletal system; pertaining to orthopaedics. [EU]

Tetanus: A disease caused by tetanospasmin, a powerful protein toxin produced by clostridium tetani. Tetanus usually occurs after an acute injury, such as a puncture wound or laceration. Generalized tetanus, the most common form, is characterized by tetanic muscular contractions and hyperreflexia. Localized tetanus presents itself as a mild condition with manifestations restricted to muscles near the wound. It may progress to the generalized form. [NIH]

Tuberculosis: Any of the infectious diseases of man and other animals caused by species of mycobacterium. [NIH]

Ventilation: 1. in respiratory physiology, the process of exchange of air between the lungs and the ambient air. Pulmonary ventilation (usually measured in litres per minute) refers to the total exchange, whereas alveolar ventilation refers to the effective ventilation of the alveoli, in which gas exchange with the blood takes place. 2. in psychiatry, verbalization of one's emotional problems. [EU]

CHAPTER   5.   MULTIMEDIA   ON   ACANTHAMOEBA INFECTION

Overview

Information on Acanthamoeba infection can come in a variety of formats. Among multimedia sources, video productions, slides, audiotapes, and computer databases are often available. In this chapter, we show you how to keep current on multimedia sources of information on Acanthamoeba infection. We start with sources that have been summarized by federal agencies, and then show you how to find bibliographic information catalogued by the National Library of Medicine. If you see an interesting item, visit your local medical library to check on the availability of the title.

Bibliography: Multimedia on Acanthamoeba Infection

The National Library of Medicine is a rich source of information on healthcare-related multimedia productions including slides, computer software, and databases. To access the multimedia database, go to the following Web site: **http://locatorplus.gov/**. Select "Search LOCATORplus." Once in the search area, simply type in Acanthamoeba infection (or synonyms). Then, in the option box provided below the search box, select "Audiovisuals and Computer Files." From there, you can choose to sort results by publication date, author, or relevance. The following multimedia has been indexed on Acanthamoeba infection. For more information, follow the hyperlink indicated:

- **Avoidance of complications from major oncologic procedures.** Source: SSO, the Society of Surgical Oncology, 52nd Annual Cancer Symposium,

March 4-7, 1999, Orlando, FL; Year: 1999; Format: Videorecording; [Chicago, Ill.]: Distributed by Teach'em, [1999]

- **Infection control : break the chain.** Source: Coastal Health+Train; produced by Coastal Training Technologies Corp; Year: 1999; Format: Videorecording; Virginia Beach, VA: The Corp., c1999

- **Infection control and standard precautions: new guidelines for healthcare workers.** Source: [presented] by Medcom; Year: 1997; Format: Videorecording; Cypress, CA: Medcom, c1992 [i.e. c1997]

- **Infection control for ambulatory care.** Source: Coastal Health+Train; produced by Coastal Training Technologies; Year: 2000; Format: Videorecording; Virginia Beach, VA: Coastal Training Technologies Corp., c2000

- **Infection control in home healthcare: winning the battle.** Source: Coastal Health+Train; produced by Coastal Training Technologies Corp; Year: 1998; Format: Videorecording; Virginia Beach, VA: The Corporation, c1998

- **Protect yourself: preventing infectious disease transmitted by blood, body fluids, and tissue.** Source: NCCLS; Year: 1998; Format: Videorecording; Wayne, PA: NCCLS, c1998

- **Safety in healthcare: infection control.** Source: produced by J.J. Keller & Associates, Inc; Year: 2000; Format: Videorecording; Neenah, WI: J.J. Keller; Associates, c2000

Vocabulary Builder

Asepsis: 1. freedom from infection. 2. the prevention of contact with microorganisms. [EU]

Catheterization: The employment or passage of a catheter. [EU]

Perioperative: Pertaining to the period extending from the time of hospitalization for surgery to the time of discharge. [EU]

CHAPTER 6. PHYSICIAN GUIDELINES AND DATABASES

Overview

Doctors and medical researchers rely on a number of information sources to help patients with their conditions. Many will subscribe to journals or newsletters published by their professional associations or refer to specialized textbooks or clinical guides published for the medical profession. In this chapter, we focus on databases and Internet-based guidelines created or written for this professional audience.

NIH Guidelines

For the more common diseases, The National Institutes of Health publish guidelines that are frequently consulted by physicians. Publications are typically written by one or more of the various NIH Institutes. For physician guidelines, commonly referred to as "clinical" or "professional" guidelines, you can visit the following Institutes:

- Office of the Director (OD); guidelines consolidated across agencies available at **http://www.nih.gov/health/consumer/conkey.htm**

- National Institute of General Medical Sciences (NIGMS); fact sheets available at **http://www.nigms.nih.gov/news/facts/**

- National Library of Medicine (NLM); extensive encyclopedia (A.D.A.M., Inc.) with guidelines:
  http://www.nlm.nih.gov/medlineplus/healthtopics.html

- National Institute of Allergy and Infectious Diseases (NIAID); guidelines available at **http://www.niaid.nih.gov/publications/**

- Centers for Disease Control and Prevention; various fact sheets on infectious diseases available at **http://www.cdc.gov/health/diseases.htm**

NIH Databases

In addition to the various Institutes of Health that publish professional guidelines, the NIH has designed a number of databases for professionals.[22] Physician-oriented resources provide a wide variety of information related to the biomedical and health sciences, both past and present. The format of these resources varies. Searchable databases, bibliographic citations, full text articles (when available), archival collections, and images are all available. The following are referenced by the National Library of Medicine:[23]

- **Bioethics:** Access to published literature on the ethical, legal and public policy issues surrounding healthcare and biomedical research. This information is provided in conjunction with the Kennedy Institute of Ethics located at Georgetown University, Washington, D.C.: **http://www.nlm.nih.gov/databases/databases_bioethics.html**

- **HIV/AIDS Resources:** Describes various links and databases dedicated to HIV/AIDS research: **http://www.nlm.nih.gov/pubs/factsheets/aidsinfs.html**

- **NLM Online Exhibitions:** Describes "Exhibitions in the History of Medicine": **http://www.nlm.nih.gov/exhibition/exhibition.html**. Additional resources for historical scholarship in medicine: **http://www.nlm.nih.gov/hmd/hmd.html**

- **Biotechnology Information:** Access to public databases. The National Center for Biotechnology Information conducts research in computational biology, develops software tools for analyzing genome data, and disseminates biomedical information for the better understanding of molecular processes affecting human health and disease: **http://www.ncbi.nlm.nih.gov/**

- **Population Information:** The National Library of Medicine provides access to worldwide coverage of population, family planning, and related health issues, including family planning technology and programs, fertility, and population law and policy: **http://www.nlm.nih.gov/databases/databases_population.html**

---

[22] Remember, for the general public, the National Library of Medicine recommends the databases referenced in MEDLINE*plus* (**http://medlineplus.gov/** or **http://www.nlm.nih.gov/medlineplus/databases.html**).
[23] See **http://www.nlm.nih.gov/databases/databases.html**.

- **Cancer Information:** Access to caner-oriented databases: http://www.nlm.nih.gov/databases/databases_cancer.html

- **Profiles in Science:** Offering the archival collections of prominent twentieth-century biomedical scientists to the public through modern digital technology: http://www.profiles.nlm.nih.gov/

- **Chemical Information:** Provides links to various chemical databases and references: http://sis.nlm.nih.gov/Chem/ChemMain.html

- **Clinical Alerts:** Reports the release of findings from the NIH-funded clinical trials where such release could significantly affect morbidity and mortality: http://www.nlm.nih.gov/databases/alerts/clinical_alerts.html

- **Space Life Sciences:** Provides links and information to space-based research (including NASA): http://www.nlm.nih.gov/databases/databases_space.html

- **MEDLINE:** Bibliographic database covering the fields of medicine, nursing, dentistry, veterinary medicine, the healthcare system, and the pre-clinical sciences: http://www.nlm.nih.gov/databases/databases_medline.html

- **Toxicology and Environmental Health Information (TOXNET):** Databases covering toxicology and environmental health: http://sis.nlm.nih.gov/Tox/ToxMain.html

- **Visible Human Interface:** Anatomically detailed, three-dimensional representations of normal male and female human bodies: http://www.nlm.nih.gov/research/visible/visible_human.html

While all of the above references may be of interest to physicians who study and treat Acanthamoeba infection, the following are particularly noteworthy.

The NLM Gateway[24]

The NLM (National Library of Medicine) Gateway is a Web-based system that lets users search simultaneously in multiple retrieval systems at the U.S. National Library of Medicine (NLM). It allows users of NLM services to initiate searches from one Web interface, providing "one-stop searching" for many of NLM's information resources or databases.[25] One target audience

---

[24] Adapted from NLM: http://gateway.nlm.nih.gov/gw/Cmd?Overview.x.
[25] The NLM Gateway is currently being developed by the Lister Hill National Center for Biomedical Communications (LHNCBC) at the National Library of Medicine (NLM) of the National Institutes of Health (NIH).

for the Gateway is the Internet user who is new to NLM's online resources and does not know what information is available or how best to search for it. This audience may include physicians and other healthcare providers, researchers, librarians, students, and, increasingly, patients, their families, and the public.[26] To use the NLM Gateway, simply go to the search site at **http://gateway.nlm.nih.gov/gw/Cmd**. Type "Acanthamoeba infection" (or synonyms) into the search box and click "Search." The results will be presented in a tabular form, indicating the number of references in each database category.

Results Summary

Category	Items Found
Journal Articles	358
Books / Periodicals / Audio Visual	0
Consumer Health	2
Meeting Abstracts	4
Other Collections	0
Total	364

HSTAT[27]

HSTAT is a free, Web-based resource that provides access to full-text documents used in healthcare decision-making.[28] HSTAT's audience includes healthcare providers, health service researchers, policy makers, insurance companies, consumers, and the information professionals who serve these groups. HSTAT provides access to a wide variety of publications, including clinical practice guidelines, quick-reference guides for clinicians, consumer health brochures, evidence reports and technology assessments from the Agency for Healthcare Research and Quality (AHRQ), as well as

---

[26] Other users may find the Gateway useful for an overall search of NLM's information resources. Some searchers may locate what they need immediately, while others will utilize the Gateway as an adjunct tool to other NLM search services such as PubMed® and MEDLINEplus®. The Gateway connects users with multiple NLM retrieval systems while also providing a search interface for its own collections. These collections include various types of information that do not logically belong in PubMed, LOCATORplus, or other established NLM retrieval systems (e.g., meeting announcements and pre-1966 journal citations). The Gateway will provide access to the information found in an increasing number of NLM retrieval systems in several phases.

[27] Adapted from HSTAT: **http://www.nlm.nih.gov/pubs/factsheets/hstat.html**

[28] The HSTAT URL is **http://hstat.nlm.nih.gov/**.

AHRQ's Put Prevention Into Practice.[29] Simply search by "Acanthamoeba infection" (or synonyms) at the following Web site: **http://text.nlm.nih.gov**.

Coffee Break: Tutorials for Biologists[30]

Some patients may wish to have access to a general healthcare site that takes a scientific view of the news and covers recent breakthroughs in biology that may one day assist physicians in developing treatments. To this end, we recommend "Coffee Break," a collection of short reports on recent biological discoveries. Each report incorporates interactive tutorials that demonstrate how bioinformatics tools are used as a part of the research process. Currently, all Coffee Breaks are written by NCBI staff.[31] Each report is about 400 words and is usually based on a discovery reported in one or more articles from recently published, peer-reviewed literature.[32] This site has new articles every few weeks, so it can be considered an online magazine of sorts, and intended for general background information. You can access the Coffee Break Web site at **http://www.ncbi.nlm.nih.gov/Coffeebreak/**.

---

[29] Other important documents in HSTAT include: the National Institutes of Health (NIH) Consensus Conference Reports and Technology Assessment Reports; the HIV/AIDS Treatment Information Service (ATIS) resource documents; the Substance Abuse and Mental Health Services Administration's Center for Substance Abuse Treatment (SAMHSA/CSAT) Treatment Improvement Protocols (TIP) and Center for Substance Abuse Prevention (SAMHSA/CSAP) Prevention Enhancement Protocols System (PEPS); the Public Health Service (PHS) Preventive Services Task Force's *Guide to Clinical Preventive Services*; the independent, nonfederal Task Force on Community Services *Guide to Community Preventive Services*; and the Health Technology Advisory Committee (HTAC) of the Minnesota Health Care Commission (MHCC) health technology evaluations.

[30] Adapted from **http://www.ncbi.nlm.nih.gov/Coffeebreak/Archive/FAQ.html**

[31] The figure that accompanies each article is frequently supplied by an expert external to NCBI, in which case the source of the figure is cited. The result is an interactive tutorial that tells a biological story.

[32] After a brief introduction that sets the work described into a broader context, the report focuses on how a molecular understanding can provide explanations of observed biology and lead to therapies for diseases. Each vignette is accompanied by a figure and hypertext links that lead to a series of pages that interactively show how NCBI tools and resources are used in the research process.

Other Commercial Databases

In addition to resources maintained by official agencies, other databases exist that are commercial ventures addressing medical professionals. Here are a few examples that may interest you:

- **CliniWeb International:** Index and table of contents to selected clinical information on the Internet; see **http://www.ohsu.edu/cliniweb/**.

- **Image Engine:** Multimedia electronic medical record system that integrates a wide range of digitized clinical images with textual data stored in the University of Pittsburgh Medical Center's MARS electronic medical record system; see the following Web site: **http://www.cml.upmc.edu/cml/imageengine/imageEngine.html**.

- **Medical World Search:** Searches full text from thousands of selected medical sites on the Internet; see **http://www.mwsearch.com/**.

- **MedWeaver:** Prototype system that allows users to search differential diagnoses for any list of signs and symptoms, to search medical literature, and to explore relevant Web sites; see **http://www.med.virginia.edu/~wmd4n/medweaver.html**.

- **Metaphrase:** Middleware component intended for use by both caregivers and medical records personnel. It converts the informal language generally used by caregivers into terms from formal, controlled vocabularies; see **http://www.lexical.com/Metaphrase.html**.

Specialized References

The following books are specialized references written for professionals interested in Acanthamoeba infection (sorted alphabetically by title, hyperlinks provide rankings, information, and reviews at Amazon.com):

- **2002 Pocket Book of Infectious Disease Therapy** by John G. Bartlett; Paperback - 348 pages, 11th edition (November 15, 2001), Lippincott, Williams & Wilkins Publishers; ISBN: 0781734320; **http://www.amazon.com/exec/obidos/ASIN/0781734320/icongroupinterna**

- **Concepts in Microbiology, Immunology, & Infectious Disease: A Review for the Usmle Step 1 (Usmle Concepts Series)** by Kapil Gupta; Paperback (May 1997), CRC Press-Parthenon Publishers; ISBN: 1850707979; **http://www.amazon.com/exec/obidos/ASIN/1850707979/icongroupinterna**

- **Current Diagnosis & Treatment in Infectious Diseases** by Walter R. Wilson (Editor), et al; Paperback - 985 pages, 1st edition (June 22, 2001), McGraw-Hill Professional Publishing; ISBN: 0838514944; http://www.amazon.com/exec/obidos/ASIN/0838514944/icongroupinterna

- **Hunter's Tropical Medicine and Emerging Infectious Diseases** by George W. Hunter (Editor), et al; Hardcover - 1192 pages, 8th edition (January 15, 2000), W B Saunders Co; ISBN: 0721662234; http://www.amazon.com/exec/obidos/ASIN/0721662234/icongroupinterna

- **Infectious Disease** by Barbara Bannister, et al; Paperback - 506 pages, 2nd edition (August 15, 2000), Blackwell Science Inc; ISBN: 0632053194; http://www.amazon.com/exec/obidos/ASIN/0632053194/icongroupinterna

- **Infectious Disease Epidemiology: Theory and Practice** by Kenrad E. Nelson, et al; Hardcover - 600 pages (May 2000), Aspen Publishers, Inc.; ISBN: 083421766X; http://www.amazon.com/exec/obidos/ASIN/083421766X/icongroupinterna

- **Infectious Diseases Diagnosis : Current Status and Future Trends (Parasitology, 117)** by H. V. Smith (Editor), et al; Paperback - 218 pages (August 2000), Cambridge University Press; ISBN: 0521785073; http://www.amazon.com/exec/obidos/ASIN/0521785073/icongroupinterna

- **Infectious Diseases and Arthropods** by Jerome Goddard; Hardcover - 240 pages (November 1999), Humana Press; ISBN: 0896038254; http://www.amazon.com/exec/obidos/ASIN/0896038254/icongroupinterna

- **Mandell, Douglas, and Bennett's Principles & Practice of Infectious Diseases (2 Vol. Set)** by Gerald L. Mandell (Editor), et al; Hardcover - 3263 pages, 5th edition (June 15, 2000), Churchill Livingstone; ISBN: 044307593X; http://www.amazon.com/exec/obidos/ASIN/044307593X/icongroupinterna

- **Manual of Antibiotics and Infectious Diseases: Treatment and Prevention** by John E. Conte; Paperback - 755 pages, 9th edition (December 15, 2001), Lippincott, Williams & Wilkins Publishers; ISBN: 0781723167; http://www.amazon.com/exec/obidos/ASIN/0781723167/icongroupinterna

- **Molecular Epidemiology of Infectious Diseases** by R. C. Andrew Thompson; Hardcover - 326 pages, 1st edition (October 15, 2000), Edward Arnold; ISBN: 0340759097; http://www.amazon.com/exec/obidos/ASIN/0340759097/icongroupinterna

- **Tropical Medicine and Parasitology** by Wallace Peters, Geoffrey Pasvol; Paperback - 334 pages, 5th edition (January 15, 2002), Mosby-Year Book; ISBN: 0723431914; http://www.amazon.com/exec/obidos/ASIN/0723431914/icongroupinterna

PART III. APPENDICES

ABOUT PART III

Part III is a collection of appendices on general medical topics which may be of interest to patients with Acanthamoeba infection and related conditions.

APPENDIX A. RESEARCHING YOUR MEDICATIONS

Overview

There are a number of sources available on new or existing medications which could be prescribed to patients with Acanthamoeba infection. While a number of hard copy or CD-Rom resources are available to patients and physicians for research purposes, a more flexible method is to use Internet-based databases. In this chapter, we will begin with a general overview of medications. We will then proceed to outline official recommendations on how you should view your medications. You may also want to research medications that you are currently taking for other conditions as they may interact with medications for Acanthamoeba infection. Research can give you information on the side effects, interactions, and limitations of prescription drugs used in the treatment of Acanthamoeba infection. Broadly speaking, there are two sources of information on approved medications: public sources and private sources. We will emphasize free-to-use public sources.

Your Medications: The Basics[33]

The Agency for Health Care Research and Quality has published extremely useful guidelines on how you can best participate in the medication aspects of Acanthamoeba infection. Taking medicines is not always as simple as swallowing a pill. It can involve many steps and decisions each day. The AHCRQ recommends that patients with Acanthamoeba infection take part in treatment decisions. Do not be afraid to ask questions and talk about your concerns. By taking a moment to ask questions early, you may avoid problems later. Here are some points to cover each time a new medicine is prescribed:

- Ask about all parts of your treatment, including diet changes, exercise, and medicines.

- Ask about the risks and benefits of each medicine or other treatment you might receive.

- Ask how often you or your doctor will check for side effects from a given medication.

Do not hesitate to ask what is important to you about your medicines. You may want a medicine with the fewest side effects, or the fewest doses to take each day. You may care most about cost, or how the medicine might affect how you live or work. Or, you may want the medicine your doctor believes will work the best. Telling your doctor will help him or her select the best treatment for you.

Do not be afraid to "bother" your doctor with your concerns and questions about medications for Acanthamoeba infection. You can also talk to a nurse or a pharmacist. They can help you better understand your treatment plan. Feel free to bring a friend or family member with you when you visit your doctor. Talking over your options with someone you trust can help you make better choices, especially if you are not feeling well. Specifically, ask your doctor the following:

- The name of the medicine and what it is supposed to do.

- How and when to take the medicine, how much to take, and for how long.

- What food, drinks, other medicines, or activities you should avoid while taking the medicine.

- What side effects the medicine may have, and what to do if they occur.

---

[33] This section is adapted from AHCRQ: **http://www.ahcpr.gov/consumer/ncpiebro.htm**.

- If you can get a refill, and how often.

- About any terms or directions you do not understand.

- What to do if you miss a dose.

- If there is written information you can take home (most pharmacies have information sheets on your prescription medicines; some even offer large-print or Spanish versions).

Do not forget to tell your doctor about all the medicines you are currently taking (not just those for Acanthamoeba infection). This includes prescription medicines and the medicines that you buy over the counter. Then your doctor can avoid giving you a new medicine that may not work well with the medications you take now. When talking to your doctor, you may wish to prepare a list of medicines you currently take, the reason you take them, and how you take them. Be sure to include the following information for each:

- Name of medicine

- Reason taken

- Dosage

- Time(s) of day

Also include any over-the-counter medicines, such as:

- Laxatives

- Diet pills

- Vitamins

- Cold medicine

- Aspirin or other pain, headache, or fever medicine

- Cough medicine

- Allergy relief medicine

- Antacids

- Sleeping pills

- Others (include names)

Learning More about Your Medications

Because of historical investments by various organizations and the emergence of the Internet, it has become rather simple to learn about the medications your doctor has recommended for Acanthamoeba infection. One such source is the United States Pharmacopeia. In 1820, eleven physicians met in Washington, D.C. to establish the first compendium of standard drugs for the United States. They called this compendium the "U.S. Pharmacopeia (USP)." Today, the USP is a non-profit organization consisting of 800 volunteer scientists, eleven elected officials, and 400 representatives of state associations and colleges of medicine and pharmacy. The USP is located in Rockville, Maryland, and its home page is located at **www.usp.org**. The USP currently provides standards for over 3,700 medications. The resulting USP DI® Advice for the Patient® can be accessed through the National Library of Medicine of the National Institutes of Health. The database is partially derived from lists of federally approved medications in the Food and Drug Administration's (FDA) Drug Approvals database.[34]

While the FDA database is rather large and difficult to navigate, the Phamacopeia is both user-friendly and free to use. It covers more than 9,000 prescription and over-the-counter medications. To access this database, simply type the following hyperlink into your Web browser: **http://www.nlm.nih.gov/medlineplus/druginformation.html**. To view examples of a given medication (brand names, category, description, preparation, proper use, precautions, side effects, etc.), simply follow the hyperlinks indicated within the United States Pharmacopoeia (USP). It is important to read the disclaimer by the USP (**http://www.nlm.nih.gov/medlineplus/drugdisclaimer.html**) before using the information provided.

Commercial Databases

In addition to the medications listed in the USP above, a number of commercial sites are available by subscription to physicians and their institutions. You may be able to access these sources from your local medical library or your doctor's office.

---

[34] Though cumbersome, the FDA database can be freely browsed at the following site: **www.fda.gov/cder/da/da.htm**.

Reuters Health Drug Database

The Reuters Health Drug Database can be searched by keyword at the hyperlink: **http://www.reutershealth.com/frame2/drug.html**. The following medications are listed in the Reuters' database as associated with Acanthamoeba infection (including those with contraindications):[35]

- **Bimatoprost**
  http://www.reutershealth.com/atoz/html/Bimatoprost.htm

- **Chloramphenicol**
  http://www.reutershealth.com/atoz/html/Chloramphenicol.htm

- **Ciprofloxacin**
  http://www.reutershealth.com/atoz/html/Ciprofloxacin.htm

- **Dexamethasone**
  http://www.reutershealth.com/atoz/html/Dexamethasone.htm

- **Dorzolamide**
  http://www.reutershealth.com/atoz/html/Dorzolamide.htm

- **Erythromycin**
  http://www.reutershealth.com/atoz/html/Erythromycin.htm

- **Flurbiprofen**
  http://www.reutershealth.com/atoz/html/Flurbiprofen.htm

- **Gentamicin**
  http://www.reutershealth.com/atoz/html/Gentamicin.htm

- **Idoxuridine (IDU)**
  http://www.reutershealth.com/atoz/html/Idoxuridine_(IDU).htm

- **Natamycin**
  http://www.reutershealth.com/atoz/html/Natamycin.htm

- **Norfloxacin**
  http://www.reutershealth.com/atoz/html/Norfloxacin.htm

- **Ofloxacin**
  http://www.reutershealth.com/atoz/html/Ofloxacin.htm

- **Prednisolone**
  http://www.reutershealth.com/atoz/html/Prednisolone.htm

- **Tetracycline HCl**
  http://www.reutershealth.com/atoz/html/Tetracycline_HCl.htm

---

[35] Adapted from *A to Z Drug Facts* by Facts and Comparisons.

- **Tobramycin**
  http://www.reutershealth.com/atoz/html/Tobramycin.htm
- **Travoprost**
  http://www.reutershealth.com/atoz/html/Travoprost.htm
- **Unoprostone Isopropyl**
  http://www.reutershealth.com/atoz/html/Unoprostone_Isopropyl.htm

Mosby's GenRx

Mosby's GenRx database (also available on CD-Rom and book format) covers 45,000 drug products including generics and international brands. It provides prescribing information, drug interactions, and patient information. Information can be obtained at the following hyperlink: **http://www.genrx.com/Mosby/PhyGenRx/group.html**.

Physicians Desk Reference

The Physicians Desk Reference database (also available in CD-Rom and book format) is a full-text drug database. The database is searchable by brand name, generic name or by indication. It features multiple drug interactions reports. Information can be obtained at the following hyperlink: **http://physician.pdr.net/physician/templates/en/acl/psuser_t.htm**.

Other Web Sites

A number of additional Web sites discuss drug information. As an example, you may like to look at **www.drugs.com** which reproduces the information in the Pharmacopeia as well as commercial information. You may also want to consider the Web site of the Medical Letter, Inc. which allows users to download articles on various drugs and therapeutics for a nominal fee: **http://www.medletter.com/**.

Contraindications and Interactions (Hidden Dangers)

Some of the medications mentioned in the previous discussions can be problematic for patients with Acanthamoeba infection--not because they are used in the treatment process, but because of contraindications, or side effects. Medications with contraindications are those that could react with drugs used to treat Acanthamoeba infection or potentially create deleterious side effects in patients with Acanthamoeba infection. You should ask your physician about any contraindications, especially as these might apply to other medications that you may be taking for common ailments.

Drug-drug interactions occur when two or more drugs react with each other. This drug-drug interaction may cause you to experience an unexpected side effect. Drug interactions may make your medications less effective, cause unexpected side effects, or increase the action of a particular drug. Some drug interactions can even be harmful to you.

Be sure to read the label every time you use a nonprescription or prescription drug, and take the time to learn about drug interactions. These precautions may be critical to your health. You can reduce the risk of potentially harmful drug interactions and side effects with a little bit of knowledge and common sense.

Drug labels contain important information about ingredients, uses, warnings, and directions which you should take the time to read and understand. Labels also include warnings about possible drug interactions. Further, drug labels may change as new information becomes available. This is why it's especially important to read the label every time you use a medication. When your doctor prescribes a new drug, discuss all over-the-counter and prescription medications, dietary supplements, vitamins, botanicals, minerals and herbals you take as well as the foods you eat. Ask your pharmacist for the package insert for each prescription drug you take. The package insert provides more information about potential drug interactions.

A Final Warning

At some point, you may hear of alternative medications from friends, relatives, or in the news media. Advertisements may suggest that certain alternative drugs can produce positive results for patients with Acanthamoeba infection. Exercise caution--some of these drugs may have fraudulent claims, and others may actually hurt you. The Food and Drug Administration (FDA) is the official U.S. agency charged with discovering which medications are likely to improve the health of patients with Acanthamoeba infection. The FDA warns patients to watch out for[36]:

- Secret formulas (real scientists share what they know)

---

[36] This section has been adapted from **http://www.fda.gov/opacom/lowlit/medfraud.html**

- Amazing breakthroughs or miracle cures (real breakthroughs don't happen very often; when they do, real scientists do not call them amazing or miracles)

- Quick, painless, or guaranteed cures

- If it sounds too good to be true, it probably isn't true.

If you have any questions about any kind of medical treatment, the FDA may have an office near you. Look for their number in the blue pages of the phone book. You can also contact the FDA through its toll-free number, 1-888-INFO-FDA (1-888-463-6332), or on the World Wide Web at **www.fda.gov**.

General References

In addition to the resources provided earlier in this chapter, the following general references describe medications (sorted alphabetically by title; hyperlinks provide rankings, information and reviews at Amazon.com):

- **Approaches to Design and Synthesis of Antiparasitic Drugs** by Satyavan Sharma, et al; Hardcover - 524 pages (October 1, 1997), Elsevier Science; ISBN: 0444894764; **http://www.amazon.com/exec/obidos/ASIN/0444894764/icongroupinterna**

- **Drug Interactions in Infectious Diseases (Infectious Disease)** by Stephen C. Piscitelli (Editor), et al; Hardcover - 372 pages (September 2000), Humana Press; ISBN: 0896037509; **http://www.amazon.com/exec/obidos/ASIN/0896037509/icongroupinterna**

- **Management of Antimicrobials in Infectious Diseases: Impact of Antibiotic Resistance** by Arch G. Mainous, Ph.D. (Editor), et al; Hardcover - 350 pages, 1st edition (January 15, 2001), Humana Press; ISBN: 0896038211; **http://www.amazon.com/exec/obidos/ASIN/0896038211/icongroupinterna**

APPENDIX B. FINDING MEDICAL LIBRARIES

Overview

At a medical library you can find medical texts and reference books, consumer health publications, specialty newspapers and magazines, as well as medical journals. In this Appendix, we show you how to quickly find a medical library in your area.

Preparation

Before going to the library, highlight the references mentioned in this sourcebook that you find interesting. Focus on those items that are not available via the Internet, and ask the reference librarian for help with your search. He or she may know of additional resources that could be helpful to you. Most importantly, your local public library and medical libraries have Interlibrary Loan programs with the National Library of Medicine (NLM), one of the largest medical collections in the world. According to the NLM, most of the literature in the general and historical collections of the National Library of Medicine is available on interlibrary loan to any library. NLM's interlibrary loan services are only available to libraries. If you would like to access NLM medical literature, then visit a library in your area that can request the publications for you.[37]

---

[37] Adapted from the NLM: **http://www.nlm.nih.gov/psd/cas/interlibrary.html**

Finding a Local Medical Library

The quickest method to locate medical libraries is to use the Internet-based directory published by the National Network of Libraries of Medicine (NN/LM). This network includes 4626 members and affiliates that provide many services to librarians, health professionals, and the public. To find a library in your area, simply visit **http://nnlm.gov/members/adv.html** or call 1-800-338-7657.

Medical Libraries Open to the Public

In addition to the NN/LM, the National Library of Medicine (NLM) lists a number of libraries that are generally open to the public and have reference facilities. The following is the NLM's list plus hyperlinks to each library Web site. These Web pages can provide information on hours of operation and other restrictions. The list below is a small sample of libraries recommended by the National Library of Medicine (sorted alphabetically by name of the U.S. state or Canadian province where the library is located):[38]

- **Alabama:** Health InfoNet of Jefferson County (Jefferson County Library Cooperative, Lister Hill Library of the Health Sciences), **http://www.uab.edu/infonet/**

- **Alabama:** Richard M. Scrushy Library (American Sports Medicine Institute), **http://www.asmi.org/LIBRARY.HTM**

- **Arizona:** Samaritan Regional Medical Center: The Learning Center (Samaritan Health System, Phoenix, Arizona), **http://www.samaritan.edu/library/bannerlibs.htm**

- **California:** Kris Kelly Health Information Center (St. Joseph Health System), **http://www.humboldt1.com/~kkhic/index.html**

- **California:** Community Health Library of Los Gatos (Community Health Library of Los Gatos), **http://www.healthlib.org/orgresources.html**

- **California:** Consumer Health Program and Services (CHIPS) (County of Los Angeles Public Library, Los Angeles County Harbor-UCLA Medical Center Library) - Carson, CA, **http://www.colapublib.org/services/chips.html**

- **California:** Gateway Health Library (Sutter Gould Medical Foundation)

- **California:** Health Library (Stanford University Medical Center), **http://www-med.stanford.edu/healthlibrary/**

---

[38] Abstracted from **http://www.nlm.nih.gov/medlineplus/libraries.html**

- **California:** Patient Education Resource Center - Health Information and Resources (University of California, San Francisco), **http://sfghdean.ucsf.edu/barnett/PERC/default.asp**

- **California:** Redwood Health Library (Petaluma Health Care District), **http://www.phcd.org/rdwdlib.html**

- **California:** San José PlaneTree Health Library, **http://planetreesanjose.org/**

- **California:** Sutter Resource Library (Sutter Hospitals Foundation), **http://go.sutterhealth.org/comm/resc-library/sac-resources.html**

- **California:** University of California, Davis. Health Sciences Libraries

- **California:** ValleyCare Health Library & Ryan Comer Cancer Resource Center (ValleyCare Health System), **http://www.valleycare.com/library.html**

- **California:** Washington Community Health Resource Library (Washington Community Health Resource Library), **http://www.healthlibrary.org/**

- **Colorado:** William V. Gervasini Memorial Library (Exempla Healthcare), **http://www.exempla.org/conslib.htm**

- **Connecticut:** Hartford Hospital Health Science Libraries (Hartford Hospital), **http://www.harthosp.org/library/**

- **Connecticut:** Healthnet: Connecticut Consumer Health Information Center (University of Connecticut Health Center, Lyman Maynard Stowe Library), **http://library.uchc.edu/departm/hnet/**

- **Connecticut:** Waterbury Hospital Health Center Library (Waterbury Hospital), **http://www.waterburyhospital.com/library/consumer.shtml**

- **Delaware:** Consumer Health Library (Christiana Care Health System, Eugene du Pont Preventive Medicine & Rehabilitation Institute), **http://www.christianacare.org/health_guide/health_guide_pmri_health _info.cfm**

- **Delaware:** Lewis B. Flinn Library (Delaware Academy of Medicine), **http://www.delamed.org/chls.html**

- **Georgia:** Family Resource Library (Medical College of Georgia), **http://cmc.mcg.edu/kids_families/fam_resources/fam_res_lib/frl.htm**

- **Georgia:** Health Resource Center (Medical Center of Central Georgia), **http://www.mccg.org/hrc/hrchome.asp**

- **Hawaii:** Hawaii Medical Library: Consumer Health Information Service (Hawaii Medical Library), **http://hml.org/CHIS/**

- **Idaho:** DeArmond Consumer Health Library (Kootenai Medical Center), http://www.nicon.org/DeArmond/index.htm

- **Illinois:** Health Learning Center of Northwestern Memorial Hospital (Northwestern Memorial Hospital, Health Learning Center), http://www.nmh.org/health_info/hlc.html

- **Illinois:** Medical Library (OSF Saint Francis Medical Center), http://www.osfsaintfrancis.org/general/library/

- **Kentucky:** Medical Library - Services for Patients, Families, Students & the Public (Central Baptist Hospital), http://www.centralbap.com/education/community/library.htm

- **Kentucky:** University of Kentucky - Health Information Library (University of Kentucky, Chandler Medical Center, Health Information Library), http://www.mc.uky.edu/PatientEd/

- **Louisiana:** Alton Ochsner Medical Foundation Library (Alton Ochsner Medical Foundation), http://www.ochsner.org/library/

- **Louisiana:** Louisiana State University Health Sciences Center Medical Library-Shreveport, http://lib-sh.lsuhsc.edu/

- **Maine:** Franklin Memorial Hospital Medical Library (Franklin Memorial Hospital), http://www.fchn.org/fmh/lib.htm

- **Maine:** Gerrish-True Health Sciences Library (Central Maine Medical Center), http://www.cmmc.org/library/library.html

- **Maine:** Hadley Parrot Health Science Library (Eastern Maine Healthcare), http://www.emh.org/hll/hpl/guide.htm

- **Maine:** Maine Medical Center Library (Maine Medical Center), http://www.mmc.org/library/

- **Maine:** Parkview Hospital, http://www.parkviewhospital.org/communit.htm#Library

- **Maine:** Southern Maine Medical Center Health Sciences Library (Southern Maine Medical Center), http://www.smmc.org/services/service.php3?choice=10

- **Maine:** Stephens Memorial Hospital Health Information Library (Western Maine Health), http://www.wmhcc.com/hil_frame.html

- **Manitoba, Canada:** Consumer & Patient Health Information Service (University of Manitoba Libraries), http://www.umanitoba.ca/libraries/units/health/reference/chis.html

- **Manitoba, Canada:** J.W. Crane Memorial Library (Deer Lodge Centre), http://www.deerlodge.mb.ca/library/libraryservices.shtml

- **Maryland:** Health Information Center at the Wheaton Regional Library (Montgomery County, Md., Dept. of Public Libraries, Wheaton Regional Library), **http://www.mont.lib.md.us/healthinfo/hic.asp**

- **Massachusetts:** Baystate Medical Center Library (Baystate Health System), **http://www.baystatehealth.com/1024/**

- **Massachusetts:** Boston University Medical Center Alumni Medical Library (Boston University Medical Center), **http://med-libwww.bu.edu/library/lib.html**

- **Massachusetts:** Lowell General Hospital Health Sciences Library (Lowell General Hospital), **http://www.lowellgeneral.org/library/HomePageLinks/WWW.htm**

- **Massachusetts:** Paul E. Woodard Health Sciences Library (New England Baptist Hospital), **http://www.nebh.org/health_lib.asp**

- **Massachusetts:** St. Luke's Hospital Health Sciences Library (St. Luke's Hospital), **http://www.southcoast.org/library/**

- **Massachusetts:** Treadwell Library Consumer Health Reference Center (Massachusetts General Hospital), **http://www.mgh.harvard.edu/library/chrcindex.html**

- **Massachusetts:** UMass HealthNet (University of Massachusetts Medical School), **http://healthnet.umassmed.edu/**

- **Michigan:** Botsford General Hospital Library - Consumer Health (Botsford General Hospital, Library & Internet Services), **http://www.botsfordlibrary.org/consumer.htm**

- **Michigan:** Helen DeRoy Medical Library (Providence Hospital and Medical Centers), **http://www.providence-hospital.org/library/**

- **Michigan:** Marquette General Hospital - Consumer Health Library (Marquette General Hospital, Health Information Center), **http://www.mgh.org/center.html**

- **Michigan:** Patient Education Resouce Center - University of Michigan Cancer Center (University of Michigan Comprehensive Cancer Center), **http://www.cancer.med.umich.edu/learn/leares.htm**

- **Michigan:** Sladen Library & Center for Health Information Resources - Consumer Health Information, **http://www.sladen.hfhs.org/library/consumer/index.html**

- **Montana:** Center for Health Information (St. Patrick Hospital and Health Sciences Center), **http://www.saintpatrick.org/chi/librarydetail.php3?ID=41**

- **National:** Consumer Health Library Directory (Medical Library Association, Consumer and Patient Health Information Section), **http://caphis.mlanet.org/directory/index.html**

- **National:** National Network of Libraries of Medicine (National Library of Medicine) - provides library services for health professionals in the United States who do not have access to a medical library, **http://nnlm.gov/**

- **National:** NN/LM List of Libraries Serving the Public (National Network of Libraries of Medicine), **http://nnlm.gov/members/**

- **Nevada:** Health Science Library, West Charleston Library (Las Vegas Clark County Library District), **http://www.lvccld.org/special_collections/medical/index.htm**

- **New Hampshire:** Dartmouth Biomedical Libraries (Dartmouth College Library), **http://www.dartmouth.edu/~biomed/resources.htmld/conshealth.htmld/**

- **New Jersey:** Consumer Health Library (Rahway Hospital), **http://www.rahwayhospital.com/library.htm**

- **New Jersey:** Dr. Walter Phillips Health Sciences Library (Englewood Hospital and Medical Center), **http://www.englewoodhospital.com/links/index.htm**

- **New Jersey:** Meland Foundation (Englewood Hospital and Medical Center), **http://www.geocities.com/ResearchTriangle/9360/**

- **New York:** Choices in Health Information (New York Public Library) - NLM Consumer Pilot Project participant, **http://www.nypl.org/branch/health/links.html**

- **New York:** Health Information Center (Upstate Medical University, State University of New York), **http://www.upstate.edu/library/hic/**

- **New York:** Health Sciences Library (Long Island Jewish Medical Center), **http://www.lij.edu/library/library.html**

- **New York:** ViaHealth Medical Library (Rochester General Hospital), **http://www.nyam.org/library/**

- **Ohio:** Consumer Health Library (Akron General Medical Center, Medical & Consumer Health Library), **http://www.akrongeneral.org/hwlibrary.htm**

- **Oklahoma:** Saint Francis Health System Patient/Family Resource Center (Saint Francis Health System), **http://www.sfh-tulsa.com/patientfamilycenter/default.asp**

- **Oregon:** Planetree Health Resource Center (Mid-Columbia Medical Center), **http://www.mcmc.net/phrc/**

- **Pennsylvania:** Community Health Information Library (Milton S. Hershey Medical Center), **http://www.hmc.psu.edu/commhealth/**

- **Pennsylvania:** Community Health Resource Library (Geisinger Medical Center), **http://www.geisinger.edu/education/commlib.shtml**

- **Pennsylvania:** HealthInfo Library (Moses Taylor Hospital), **http://www.mth.org/healthwellness.html**

- **Pennsylvania:** Hopwood Library (University of Pittsburgh, Health Sciences Library System), **http://www.hsls.pitt.edu/chi/hhrcinfo.html**

- **Pennsylvania:** Koop Community Health Information Center (College of Physicians of Philadelphia), **http://www.collphyphil.org/kooppg1.shtml**

- **Pennsylvania:** Learning Resources Center - Medical Library (Susquehanna Health System), **http://www.shscares.org/services/lrc/index.asp**

- **Pennsylvania:** Medical Library (UPMC Health System), **http://www.upmc.edu/passavant/library.htm**

- **Quebec, Canada:** Medical Library (Montreal General Hospital), **http://ww2.mcgill.ca/mghlib/**

- **South Dakota:** Rapid City Regional Hospital - Health Information Center (Rapid City Regional Hospital, Health Information Center), **http://www.rcrh.org/education/LibraryResourcesConsumers.htm**

- **Texas:** Houston HealthWays (Houston Academy of Medicine-Texas Medical Center Library), **http://hhw.library.tmc.edu/**

- **Texas:** Matustik Family Resource Center (Cook Children's Health Care System), **http://www.cookchildrens.com/Matustik_Library.html**

- **Washington:** Community Health Library (Kittitas Valley Community Hospital), **http://www.kvch.com/**

- **Washington:** Southwest Washington Medical Center Library (Southwest Washington Medical Center), **http://www.swmedctr.com/Home/**

APPENDIX C. YOUR RIGHTS AND INSURANCE

Overview

Any patient with Acanthamoeba infection faces a series of issues related more to the healthcare industry than to the medical condition itself. This appendix covers two important topics in this regard: your rights and responsibilities as a patient, and how to get the most out of your medical insurance plan.

Your Rights as a Patient

The President's Advisory Commission on Consumer Protection and Quality in the Healthcare Industry has created the following summary of your rights as a patient.[39]

Information Disclosure

Consumers have the right to receive accurate, easily understood information. Some consumers require assistance in making informed decisions about health plans, health professionals, and healthcare facilities. Such information includes:

- *Health plans.* Covered benefits, cost-sharing, and procedures for resolving complaints, licensure, certification, and accreditation status, comparable measures of quality and consumer satisfaction, provider

---

[39]Adapted from Consumer Bill of Rights and Responsibilities:
http://www.hcqualitycommission.gov/press/cbor.html#head1.

network composition, the procedures that govern access to specialists and emergency services, and care management information.

- *Health professionals.* Education, board certification, and recertification, years of practice, experience performing certain procedures, and comparable measures of quality and consumer satisfaction.

- *Healthcare facilities.* Experience in performing certain procedures and services, accreditation status, comparable measures of quality, worker, and consumer satisfaction, and procedures for resolving complaints.

- *Consumer assistance programs.* Programs must be carefully structured to promote consumer confidence and to work cooperatively with health plans, providers, payers, and regulators. Desirable characteristics of such programs are sponsorship that ensures accountability to the interests of consumers and stable, adequate funding.

Choice of Providers and Plans

Consumers have the right to a choice of healthcare providers that is sufficient to ensure access to appropriate high-quality healthcare. To ensure such choice, the Commission recommends the following:

- *Provider network adequacy.* All health plan networks should provide access to sufficient numbers and types of providers to assure that all covered services will be accessible without unreasonable delay -- including access to emergency services 24 hours a day and 7 days a week. If a health plan has an insufficient number or type of providers to provide a covered benefit with the appropriate degree of specialization, the plan should ensure that the consumer obtains the benefit outside the network at no greater cost than if the benefit were obtained from participating providers.

- *Women's health services.* Women should be able to choose a qualified provider offered by a plan -- such as gynecologists, certified nurse midwives, and other qualified healthcare providers -- for the provision of covered care necessary to provide routine and preventative women's healthcare services.

- *Access to specialists.* Consumers with complex or serious medical conditions who require frequent specialty care should have direct access to a qualified specialist of their choice within a plan's network of providers. Authorizations, when required, should be for an adequate number of direct access visits under an approved treatment plan.

- *Transitional care.* Consumers who are undergoing a course of treatment for a chronic or disabling condition (or who are in the second or third trimester of a pregnancy) at the time they involuntarily change health plans or at a time when a provider is terminated by a plan for other than cause should be able to continue seeing their current specialty providers for up to 90 days (or through completion of postpartum care) to allow for transition of care.

- *Choice of health plans.* Public and private group purchasers should, wherever feasible, offer consumers a choice of high-quality health insurance plans.

Access to Emergency Services

Consumers have the right to access emergency healthcare services when and where the need arises. Health plans should provide payment when a consumer presents to an emergency department with acute symptoms of sufficient severity--including severe pain--such that a "prudent layperson" could reasonably expect the absence of medical attention to result in placing that consumer's health in serious jeopardy, serious impairment to bodily functions, or serious dysfunction of any bodily organ or part.

Participation in Treatment Decisions

Consumers have the right and responsibility to fully participate in all decisions related to their healthcare. Consumers who are unable to fully participate in treatment decisions have the right to be represented by parents, guardians, family members, or other conservators. Physicians and other health professionals should:

- Provide patients with sufficient information and opportunity to decide among treatment options consistent with the informed consent process.

- Discuss all treatment options with a patient in a culturally competent manner, including the option of no treatment at all.

- Ensure that persons with disabilities have effective communications with members of the health system in making such decisions.

- Discuss all current treatments a consumer may be undergoing.

- Discuss all risks, benefits, and consequences to treatment or nontreatment.

- Give patients the opportunity to refuse treatment and to express preferences about future treatment decisions.

- Discuss the use of advance directives -- both living wills and durable powers of attorney for healthcare -- with patients and their designated family members.

- Abide by the decisions made by their patients and/or their designated representatives consistent with the informed consent process.

Health plans, health providers, and healthcare facilities should:

- Disclose to consumers factors -- such as methods of compensation, ownership of or interest in healthcare facilities, or matters of conscience -- that could influence advice or treatment decisions.

- Assure that provider contracts do not contain any so-called "gag clauses" or other contractual mechanisms that restrict healthcare providers' ability to communicate with and advise patients about medically necessary treatment options.

- Be prohibited from penalizing or seeking retribution against healthcare professionals or other health workers for advocating on behalf of their patients.

Respect and Nondiscrimination

Consumers have the right to considerate, respectful care from all members of the healthcare industry at all times and under all circumstances. An environment of mutual respect is essential to maintain a quality healthcare system. To assure that right, the Commission recommends the following:

- Consumers must not be discriminated against in the delivery of healthcare services consistent with the benefits covered in their policy, or as required by law, based on race, ethnicity, national origin, religion, sex, age, mental or physical disability, sexual orientation, genetic information, or source of payment.

- Consumers eligible for coverage under the terms and conditions of a health plan or program, or as required by law, must not be discriminated against in marketing and enrollment practices based on race, ethnicity, national origin, religion, sex, age, mental or physical disability, sexual orientation, genetic information, or source of payment.

Confidentiality of Health Information

Consumers have the right to communicate with healthcare providers in confidence and to have the confidentiality of their individually identifiable healthcare information protected. Consumers also have the right to review and copy their own medical records and request amendments to their records.

Complaints and Appeals

Consumers have the right to a fair and efficient process for resolving differences with their health plans, healthcare providers, and the institutions that serve them, including a rigorous system of internal review and an independent system of external review. A free copy of the Patient's Bill of Rights is available from the American Hospital Association.[40]

Patient Responsibilities

Treatment is a two-way street between you and your healthcare providers. To underscore the importance of finance in modern healthcare as well as your responsibility for the financial aspects of your care, the President's Advisory Commission on Consumer Protection and Quality in the Healthcare Industry has proposed that patients understand the following "Consumer Responsibilities."[41] In a healthcare system that protects consumers' rights, it is reasonable to expect and encourage consumers to assume certain responsibilities. Greater individual involvement by the consumer in his or her care increases the likelihood of achieving the best outcome and helps support a quality-oriented, cost-conscious environment. Such responsibilities include:

- Take responsibility for maximizing healthy habits such as exercising, not smoking, and eating a healthy diet.

- Work collaboratively with healthcare providers in developing and carrying out agreed-upon treatment plans.

- Disclose relevant information and clearly communicate wants and needs.

---

[40] To order your free copy of the Patient's Bill of Rights, telephone 312-422-3000 or visit the American Hospital Association's Web site: **http://www.aha.org**. Click on "Resource Center," go to "Search" at bottom of page, and then type in "Patient's Bill of Rights." The Patient's Bill of Rights is also available from Fax on Demand, at 312-422-2020, document number 471124.

[41] Adapted from **http://www.hcqualitycommission.gov/press/cbor.html#head1**.

- Use your health insurance plan's internal complaint and appeal processes to address your concerns.

- Avoid knowingly spreading disease.

- Recognize the reality of risks, the limits of the medical science, and the human fallibility of the healthcare professional.

- Be aware of a healthcare provider's obligation to be reasonably efficient and equitable in providing care to other patients and the community.

- Become knowledgeable about your health plan's coverage and options (when available) including all covered benefits, limitations, and exclusions, rules regarding use of network providers, coverage and referral rules, appropriate processes to secure additional information, and the process to appeal coverage decisions.

- Show respect for other patients and health workers.

- Make a good-faith effort to meet financial obligations.

- Abide by administrative and operational procedures of health plans, healthcare providers, and Government health benefit programs.

Choosing an Insurance Plan

There are a number of official government agencies that help consumers understand their healthcare insurance choices.[42] The U.S. Department of Labor, in particular, recommends ten ways to make your health benefits choices work best for you.[43]

1. Your options are important. There are many different types of health benefit plans. Find out which one your employer offers, then check out the plan, or plans, offered. Your employer's human resource office, the health plan administrator, or your union can provide information to help you match your needs and preferences with the available plans. The more information you have, the better your healthcare decisions will be.

2. Reviewing the benefits available. Do the plans offered cover preventive care, well-baby care, vision or dental care? Are there deductibles? Answers to these questions can help determine the out-of-pocket expenses you may

---

[42] More information about quality across programs is provided at the following AHRQ Web site:
http://www.ahrq.gov/consumer/qntascii/qnthplan.htm .
[43] Adapted from the Department of Labor:
http://www.dol.gov/dol/pwba/public/pubs/health/top10-text.html.

face. Matching your needs and those of your family members will result in the best possible benefits. Cheapest may not always be best. Your goal is high quality health benefits.

3. Look for quality. The quality of healthcare services varies, but quality can be measured. You should consider the quality of healthcare in deciding among the healthcare plans or options available to you. Not all health plans, doctors, hospitals and other providers give the highest quality care. Fortunately, there is quality information you can use right now to help you compare your healthcare choices. Find out how you can measure quality. Consult the U.S. Department of Health and Human Services publication "Your Guide to Choosing Quality Health Care" on the Internet at **www.ahcpr.gov/consumer**.

4. Your plan's summary plan description (SPD) provides a wealth of information. Your health plan administrator can provide you with a copy of your plan's SPD. It outlines your benefits and your legal rights under the Employee Retirement Income Security Act (ERISA), the federal law that protects your health benefits. It should contain information about the coverage of dependents, what services will require a co-pay, and the circumstances under which your employer can change or terminate a health benefits plan. Save the SPD and all other health plan brochures and documents, along with memos or correspondence from your employer relating to health benefits.

5. Assess your benefit coverage as your family status changes. Marriage, divorce, childbirth or adoption, and the death of a spouse are all life events that may signal a need to change your health benefits. You, your spouse and dependent children may be eligible for a special enrollment period under provisions of the Health Insurance Portability and Accountability Act (HIPAA). Even without life-changing events, the information provided by your employer should tell you how you can change benefits or switch plans, if more than one plan is offered. If your spouse's employer also offers a health benefits package, consider coordinating both plans for maximum coverage.

6. Changing jobs and other life events can affect your health benefits. Under the Consolidated Omnibus Budget Reconciliation Act (COBRA), you, your covered spouse, and your dependent children may be eligible to purchase extended health coverage under your employer's plan if you lose your job, change employers, get divorced, or upon occurrence of certain other events. Coverage can range from 18 to 36 months depending on your situation. COBRA applies to most employers with 20 or more workers and requires your plan to notify you of your rights. Most plans require eligible individuals to make their COBRA election within 60 days of the plan's notice. Be sure to follow up with your plan sponsor if you don't receive notice, and make sure you respond within the allotted time.

7. HIPAA can also help if you are changing jobs, particularly if you have a medical condition. HIPAA generally limits pre-existing condition exclusions to a maximum of 12 months (18 months for late enrollees). HIPAA also requires this maximum period to be reduced by the length of time you had prior "creditable coverage." You should receive a certificate documenting your prior creditable coverage from your old plan when coverage ends.

8. Plan for retirement. Before you retire, find out what health benefits, if any, extend to you and your spouse during your retirement years. Consult with your employer's human resources office, your union, the plan administrator, and check your SPD. Make sure there is no conflicting information among these sources about the benefits you will receive or the circumstances under which they can change or be eliminated. With this information in hand, you can make other important choices, like finding out if you are eligible for Medicare and Medigap insurance coverage.

9. Know how to file an appeal if your health benefits claim is denied. Understand how your plan handles grievances and where to make appeals of the plan's decisions. Keep records and copies of correspondence. Check your health benefits package and your SPD to determine who is responsible for handling problems with benefit claims. Contact PWBA for customer service assistance if you are unable to obtain a response to your complaint.

10. You can take steps to improve the quality of the healthcare and the health benefits you receive. Look for and use things like Quality Reports and Accreditation Reports whenever you can. Quality reports may contain consumer ratings -- how satisfied consumers are with the doctors in their plan, for instance-- and clinical performance measures -- how well a healthcare organization prevents and treats illness. Accreditation reports provide information on how accredited organizations meet national standards, and often include clinical performance measures. Look for these quality measures whenever possible. Consult "Your Guide to Choosing Quality Health Care" on the Internet at **www.ahcpr.gov/consumer**.

Medicare and Medicaid

Illness strikes both rich and poor families. For low-income families, Medicaid is available to defer the costs of treatment. The Health Care Financing Administration (HCFA) administers Medicare, the nation's largest health insurance program, which covers 39 million Americans. In the following pages, you will learn the basics about Medicare insurance as well as useful contact information on how to find more in-depth information about Medicaid.[44]

Who is Eligible for Medicare?

Generally, you are eligible for Medicare if you or your spouse worked for at least 10 years in Medicare-covered employment and you are 65 years old and a citizen or permanent resident of the United States. You might also qualify for coverage if you are under age 65 but have a disability or End-Stage Renal disease (permanent kidney failure requiring dialysis or transplant). Here are some simple guidelines:

You can get Part A at age 65 without having to pay premiums if:

- You are already receiving retirement benefits from Social Security or the Railroad Retirement Board.

- You are eligible to receive Social Security or Railroad benefits but have not yet filed for them.

- You or your spouse had Medicare-covered government employment.

If you are under 65, you can get Part A without having to pay premiums if:

- You have received Social Security or Railroad Retirement Board disability benefit for 24 months.

- You are a kidney dialysis or kidney transplant patient.

Medicare has two parts:

- Part A (Hospital Insurance). Most people do not have to pay for Part A.

- Part B (Medical Insurance). Most people pay monthly for Part B.

---

[44] This section has been adapted from the Official U.S. Site for Medicare Information: http://www.medicare.gov/Basics/Overview.asp.

Part A (Hospital Insurance)

Helps Pay For: Inpatient hospital care, care in critical access hospitals (small facilities that give limited outpatient and inpatient services to people in rural areas) and skilled nursing facilities, hospice care, and some home healthcare.

Cost: Most people get Part A automatically when they turn age 65. You do not have to pay a monthly payment called a premium for Part A because you or a spouse paid Medicare taxes while you were working.

If you (or your spouse) did not pay Medicare taxes while you were working and you are age 65 or older, you still may be able to buy Part A. If you are not sure you have Part A, look on your red, white, and blue Medicare card. It will show "Hospital Part A" on the lower left corner of the card. You can also call the Social Security Administration toll free at 1-800-772-1213 or call your local Social Security office for more information about buying Part A. If you get benefits from the Railroad Retirement Board, call your local RRB office or 1-800-808-0772. For more information, call your Fiscal Intermediary about Part A bills and services. The phone number for the Fiscal Intermediary office in your area can be obtained from the following Web site: **http://www.medicare.gov/Contacts/home.asp**.

Part B (Medical Insurance)

Helps Pay For: Doctors, services, outpatient hospital care, and some other medical services that Part A does not cover, such as the services of physical and occupational therapists, and some home healthcare. Part B helps pay for covered services and supplies when they are medically necessary.

Cost: As of 2001, you pay the Medicare Part B premium of $50.00 per month. In some cases this amount may be higher if you did not choose Part B when you first became eligible at age 65. The cost of Part B may go up 10% for each 12-month period that you were eligible for Part B but declined coverage, except in special cases. You will have to pay the extra 10% cost for the rest of your life.

Enrolling in Part B is your choice. You can sign up for Part B anytime during a 7-month period that begins 3 months before you turn 65. Visit your local Social Security office, or call the Social Security Administration at 1-800-772-1213 to sign up. If you choose to enroll in Part B, the premium is usually taken out of your monthly Social Security, Railroad Retirement, or Civil Service Retirement payment. If you do not receive any of the above payments, Medicare sends you a bill for your part B premium every 3 months. You should receive your Medicare premium bill in the mail by the 10th of the month. If you do not, call the Social Security Administration at 1-800-772-1213, or your local Social Security office. If you get benefits from the Railroad Retirement Board, call your local RRB office or 1-800-808-0772. For more information, call your Medicare carrier about bills and services. The phone number for the Medicare carrier in your area can be found at the following Web site: **http://www.medicare.gov/Contacts/home.asp**. You may have choices in how you get your healthcare including the Original Medicare Plan, Medicare Managed Care Plans (like HMOs), and Medicare Private Fee-for-Service Plans.

Medicaid

Medicaid is a joint federal and state program that helps pay medical costs for some people with low incomes and limited resources. Medicaid programs vary from state to state. People on Medicaid may also get coverage for nursing home care and outpatient prescription drugs which are not covered by Medicare. You can find more information about Medicaid on the HCFA.gov Web site at **http://www.hcfa.gov/medicaid/medicaid.htm**.

States also have programs that pay some or all of Medicare's premiums and may also pay Medicare deductibles and coinsurance for certain people who have Medicare and a low income. To qualify, you must have:

- Part A (Hospital Insurance),

- Assets, such as bank accounts, stocks, and bonds that are not more than $4,000 for a single person, or $6,000 for a couple, and

- A monthly income that is below certain limits.

For more information on these programs, look at the Medicare Savings Programs   brochure, **http://www.medicare.gov/Library/PDFNavigation/PDFInterim.asp?Langua ge=English&Type=Pub&PubID=10126**. There are also Prescription Drug Assistance Programs available. Find information on these programs which offer discounts or free medications to individuals in need at **http://www.medicare.gov/Prescription/Home.asp**.

NORD's Medication Assistance Programs

Finally, the National Organization for Rare Disorders, Inc. (NORD) administers medication programs sponsored by humanitarian-minded pharmaceutical and biotechnology companies to help uninsured or under-insured individuals secure life-saving or life-sustaining drugs.[45] NORD programs ensure that certain vital drugs are available "to those individuals whose income is too high to qualify for Medicaid but too low to pay for their prescribed medications." The program has standards for fairness, equity, and unbiased eligibility. It currently covers some 14 programs for nine pharmaceutical companies. NORD also offers early access programs for investigational new drugs (IND) under the approved "Treatment INDs" programs of the Food and Drug Administration (FDA). In these programs, a limited number of individuals can receive investigational drugs that have yet to be approved by the FDA. These programs are generally designed for rare diseases or disorders. For more information, visit **www.rarediseases.org**.

Additional Resources

In addition to the references already listed in this chapter, you may need more information on health insurance, hospitals, or the healthcare system in general. The NIH has set up an excellent guidance Web site that addresses these and other issues. Topics include:[46]

- Health Insurance:
  http://www.nlm.nih.gov/medlineplus/healthinsurance.html

- Health Statistics:
  http://www.nlm.nih.gov/medlineplus/healthstatistics.html

- HMO and Managed Care:
  http://www.nlm.nih.gov/medlineplus/managedcare.html

- Hospice Care: **http://www.nlm.nih.gov/medlineplus/hospicecare.html**

- Medicaid: **http://www.nlm.nih.gov/medlineplus/medicaid.html**

- Medicare: **http://www.nlm.nih.gov/medlineplus/medicare.html**

- Nursing Homes and Long-term Care:
  http://www.nlm.nih.gov/medlineplus/nursinghomes.html

---

[45] Adapted from NORD: **http://www.rarediseases.org/cgi-bin/nord/progserv#patient?id=rPIzL9oD&mv_pc=30**.
[46] You can access this information at:
http://www.nlm.nih.gov/medlineplus/healthsystem.html.

- Patient's Rights, Confidentiality, Informed Consent, Ombudsman Programs, Privacy and Patient Issues:
  http://www.nlm.nih.gov/medlineplus/patientissues.html
- Veteran's Health, Persian Gulf War, Gulf War Syndrome, Agent Orange:
  http://www.nlm.nih.gov/medlineplus/veteranshealth.html

Vocabulary Builder

Antimicrobial: Killing microorganisms, or suppressing their multiplication or growth. [EU]

Ciprofloxacin: A carboxyfluoroquinoline antimicrobial agent that is effective against a wide range of microorganisms. It has been successfully and safely used in the treatment of resistant respiratory, skin, bone, joint, gastrointestinal, urinary, and genital infections. [NIH]

Erythromycin: A bacteriostatic antibiotic substance produced by Streptomyces erythreus. Erythromycin A is considered its major active component. In sensitive organisms, it inhibits protein synthesis by binding to 50S ribosomal subunits. This binding process inhibits peptidyl transferase activity and interferes with translocation of amino acids during translation and assembly of proteins. [NIH]

Flurbiprofen: An anti-inflammatory analgesic and antipyretic of the phenylalkynoic acid series. It has been shown to reduce bone resorption in periodontal disease by inhibiting carbonic anhydrase. [NIH]

Natamycin: Amphoteric macrolide antifungal antibiotic from Streptomyces natalensis or S. chattanoogensis. It is used for a variety of fungal infections, mainly topically. [NIH]

Norfloxacin: Quinoline-derived synthetic antibacterial agent with a very broad spectrum of action. Oral administration yields highly bactericidal plasma, tissue, and urine levels. Norfloxacin inhibits bacterial DNA-gyrase and is used in gastrointestinal, eye, and urinary infections. [NIH]

Prednisolone: A glucocorticoid with the general properties of the corticosteroids. It is the drug of choice for all conditions in which routine systemic corticosteroid therapy is indicated, except adrenal deficiency states. [NIH]

Tobramycin: An aminoglycoside, broad-spectrum antibiotic produced by Streptomyces tenebrarius. It is effective against gram-negative bacteria, especially the Pseudomonas species. It is a 10% component of the antibiotic complex, nebramycin, produced by the same species. [NIH]

ONLINE GLOSSARIES

The Internet provides access to a number of free-to-use medical dictionaries and glossaries. The National Library of Medicine has compiled the following list of online dictionaries:

- ADAM Medical Encyclopedia (A.D.A.M., Inc.), comprehensive medical reference: **http://www.nlm.nih.gov/medlineplus/encyclopedia.html**

- MedicineNet.com Medical Dictionary (MedicineNet, Inc.): **http://www.medterms.com/Script/Main/hp.asp**

- Merriam-Webster Medical Dictionary (Inteli-Health, Inc.): **http://www.intelihealth.com/IH/**

- Multilingual Glossary of Technical and Popular Medical Terms in Eight European Languages (European Commission) - Danish, Dutch, English, French, German, Italian, Portuguese, and Spanish: **http://allserv.rug.ac.be/~rvdstich/eugloss/welcome.html**

- On-line Medical Dictionary (CancerWEB): **http://www.graylab.ac.uk/omd/**

- Technology Glossary (National Library of Medicine) - Health Care Technology: **http://www.nlm.nih.gov/nichsr/ta101/ta10108.htm**

- Terms and Definitions (Office of Rare Diseases): **http://rarediseases.info.nih.gov/ord/glossary_a-e.html**

Beyond these, MEDLINEplus contains a very user-friendly encyclopedia covering every aspect of medicine (licensed from A.D.A.M., Inc.). The ADAM Medical Encyclopedia Web site address is **http://www.nlm.nih.gov/medlineplus/encyclopedia.html**. ADAM is also available on commercial Web sites such as Web MD (**http://my.webmd.com/adam/asset/adam_disease_articles/a_to_z/a**) and drkoop.com (**http://www.drkoop.com/**). Topics of interest can be researched by using keywords before continuing elsewhere, as these basic definitions and concepts will be useful in more advanced areas of research. You may choose to print various pages specifically relating to Acanthamoeba infection and keep them on file.

Online Dictionary Directories

The following are additional online directories compiled by the National Library of Medicine, including a number of specialized medical dictionaries and glossaries:

- Medical Dictionaries: Medical & Biological (World Health Organization):
  http://www.who.int/hlt/virtuallibrary/English/diction.htm#Medical

- MEL-Michigan Electronic Library List of Online Health and Medical Dictionaries (Michigan Electronic Library):
  http://mel.lib.mi.us/health/health-dictionaries.html

- Patient Education: Glossaries (DMOZ Open Directory Project):
  http://dmoz.org/Health/Education/Patient_Education/Glossaries/

- Web of Online Dictionaries (Bucknell University):
  http://www.yourdictionary.com/diction5.html#medicine

ACANTHAMOEBA INFECTION GLOSSARY

The following is a complete glossary of terms used in this sourcebook. The definitions are derived from official public sources including the National Institutes of Health [NIH] and the European Union [EU]. After this glossary, we list a number of additional hardbound and electronic glossaries and dictionaries that you may wish to consult.

Acanthamoeba: A genus of free-living soil amoebae that produces no flagellate stage. Its organisms are pathogens for several infections in humans and have been found in the eye, bone, brain, and respiratory tract. [NIH]

Acyclovir: Functional analog of the nucleoside guanosine. It acts as an antimetabolite, especially in viruses. It is used as an antiviral agent, especially in herpes infections. [NIH]

Antibody: An immunoglobulin molecule that has a specific amino acid sequence by virtue of which it interacts only with the antigen that induced its synthesis in cells of the lymphoid series (especially plasma cells), or with antigen closely related to it. Antibodies are classified according to their ode of action as agglutinins, bacteriolysins, haemolysins, opsonins, precipitins, etc. [EU]

Antigen: Any substance which is capable, under appropriate conditions, of inducing a specific immune response and of reacting with the products of that response, that is, with specific antibody or specifically sensitized T-lymphocytes, or both. Antigens may be soluble substances, such as toxins and foreign proteins, or particulate, such as bacteria and tissue cells; however, only the portion of the protein or polysaccharide molecule known as the antigenic determinant (q.v.) combines with antibody or a specific receptor on a lymphocyte. Abbreviated Ag. [EU]

Antimicrobial: Killing microorganisms, or suppressing their multiplication or growth. [EU]

Antiviral: Destroying viruses or suppressing their replication. [EU]

Arteries: The vessels carrying blood away from the heart. [NIH]

Asepsis: 1. freedom from infection. 2. the prevention of contact with microorganisms. [EU]

Assay: Determination of the amount of a particular constituent of a mixture, or of the biological or pharmacological potency of a drug. [EU]

Biopsy: The removal and examination, usually microscopic, of tissue from the living body, performed to establish precise diagnosis. [EU]

Bioterrorism: The use of biological agents in terrorism. This includes the malevolent use of bacteria, viruses, or toxins against people, animals, or plants. [NIH]

Cannabinoids: Compounds extracted from Cannabis sativa L. and metabolites having the cannabinoid structure. The most active constituents are tetrahydrocannabinol, cannabinol, and cannabidiol. [NIH]

Causal: Pertaining to a cause; directed against a cause. [EU]

Cerebrospinal: Pertaining to the brain and spinal cord. [EU]

Chemotaxis: The movement of cells or organisms toward or away from a substance in response to its concentration gradient. [NIH]

Chimera: An individual that contains cell populations derived from different zygotes. [NIH]

Ciprofloxacin: A carboxyfluoroquinoline antimicrobial agent that is effective against a wide range of microorganisms. It has been successfully and safely used in the treatment of resistant respiratory, skin, bone, joint, gastrointestinal, urinary, and genital infections. [NIH]

Cryptosporidium: A genus of coccidian parasites of the family cryptosporidiidae, found in the intestinal epithelium of many vertebrates including humans. [NIH]

Cyst: Any closed cavity or sac; normal or abnormal, lined by epithelium, and especially one that contains a liquid or semisolid material. [EU]

Cytokines: Non-antibody proteins secreted by inflammatory leukocytes and some non-leukocytic cells, that act as intercellular mediators. They differ from classical hormones in that they are produced by a number of tissue or cell types rather than by specialized glands. They generally act locally in a paracrine or autocrine rather than endocrine manner. [NIH]

Cytomegalovirus: A genus of the family herpesviridae, subfamily betaherpesvirinae, infecting the salivary glands, liver, spleen, lungs, eyes, and other organs, in which they produce characteristically enlarged cells with intranuclear inclusions. Infection with Cytomegalovirus is also seen as an opportunistic infection in AIDS. [NIH]

Dementia: An acquired organic mental disorder with loss of intellectual abilities of sufficient severity to interfere with social or occupational functioning. The dysfunction is multifaceted and involves memory, behavior, personality, judgment, attention, spatial relations, language, abstract thought, and other executive functions. The intellectual decline is usually progressive, and initially spares the level of consciousness. [NIH]

Diarrhea: Passage of excessively liquid or excessively frequent stools. [NIH]

Diving: An activity in which the organism plunges into water. It includes scuba and bell diving. Diving as natural behavior of animals goes here, as well as diving in decompression experiments with humans or animals. [NIH]

Electrophysiological: Pertaining to electrophysiology, that is a branch of physiology that is concerned with the electric phenomena associated with living bodies and involved in their functional activity. [EU]

Embryo: In animals, those derivatives of the fertilized ovum that eventually become the offspring, during their period of most rapid development, i.e., after the long axis appears until all major structures are represented. In man, the developing organism is an embryo from about two weeks after fertilization to the end of seventh or eighth week. [EU]

Encephalitis: Inflammation of the brain. [EU]

Epitopes: Sites on an antigen that interact with specific antibodies. [NIH]

Erythromycin: A bacteriostatic antibiotic substance produced by Streptomyces erythreus. Erythromycin A is considered its major active component. In sensitive organisms, it inhibits protein synthesis by binding to 50S ribosomal subunits. This binding process inhibits peptidyl transferase activity and interferes with translocation of amino acids during translation and assembly of proteins. [NIH]

Exogenous: Developed or originating outside the organism, as exogenous disease. [EU]

Fatal: Causing death, deadly; mortal; lethal. [EU]

Flurbiprofen: An anti-inflammatory analgesic and antipyretic of the phenylalkynoic acid series. It has been shown to reduce bone resorption in periodontal disease by inhibiting carbonic anhydrase. [NIH]

Ganglia: Clusters of multipolar neurons surrounded by a capsule of loosely organized connective tissue located outside the central nervous system. [NIH]

Genotype: The genetic constitution of the individual; the characterization of the genes. [NIH]

Gramicidin: Antibiotic mixture that is one of the two principle components of tyrothricin from Bacillus brevis. Gramicidin C or S is a cyclic, ten-amino acid polypeptide and gramicidins A, B, D, etc., seem to be linear polypeptides. The mixture is used topically for gram-positive organisms. It is toxic to blood, liver, kidneys, meninges, and the olfactory apparatus. [NIH]

Granule: A small pill made from sucrose. [EU]

Helicobacter: A genus of gram-negative, spiral-shaped bacteria that is pathogenic and has been isolated from the intestinal tract of mammals, including humans. [NIH]

Hepatitis: Inflammation of the liver. [EU]

Homologous: Corresponding in structure, position, origin, etc., as (a) the feathers of a bird and the scales of a fish, (b) antigen and its specific antibody, (c) allelic chromosomes. [EU]

Hybridization: The genetic process of crossbreeding to produce a hybrid. Hybrid nucleic acids can be formed by nucleic acid hybridization of DNA and RNA molecules. Protein hybridization allows for hybrid proteins to be formed from polypeptide chains. [NIH]

Hygienic: Pertaining to hygiene, or conducive to health. [EU]

Immunity: The condition of being immune; the protection against infectious disease conferred either by the immune response generated by immunization or previous infection or by other nonimmunologic factors (innate i.). [EU]

Immunohistochemistry: Histochemical localization of immunoreactive substances using labeled antibodies as reagents. [NIH]

Immunotherapy: Manipulation of the host's immune system in treatment of disease. It includes both active and passive immunization as well as immunosuppressive therapy to prevent graft rejection. [NIH]

Infiltration: The diffusion or accumulation in a tissue or cells of substances not normal to it or in amounts of the normal. Also, the material so accumulated. [EU]

Inflammation: A pathological process characterized by injury or destruction of tissues caused by a variety of cytologic and chemical reactions. It is usually manifested by typical signs of pain, heat, redness, swelling, and loss of function. [NIH]

Interneurons: Most generally any neurons which are not motor or sensory. Interneurons may also refer to neurons whose axons remain within a particular brain region as contrasted with projection neurons which have axons projecting to other brain regions. [NIH]

Keratitis: Inflammation of the cornea. [EU]

Kinetic: Pertaining to or producing motion. [EU]

Lenses: Pieces of glass or other transparent materials used for magnification or increased visual acuity. [NIH]

Lesion: Any pathological α traumatic discontinuity of tissue or loss of function of a part. [EU]

Lobe: A more or less well-defined portion of any organ, especially of the brain, lungs, and glands. Lobes are demarcated by fissures, sulci, connective tissue, and by their shape. [EU]

Lymphocytic: Pertaining to, characterized by, or of the nature of lymphocytes. [EU]

Mental: Pertaining to the mind; psychic. 2. (L. mentum chin) pertaining to the chin. [EU]

Microbiology: The study of microorganisms such as fungi, bacteria, algae, archaea, and viruses. [NIH]

Microscopy: The application of microscope magnification to the study of materials that cannot be properly seen by the unaided eye. [NIH]

Molecular: Of, pertaining to, or composed of molecules : a very small mass of matter. [EU]

Mononucleosis: The presence of an abnormally large number of mononuclear leucocytes (monocytes) in the blood. The term is often used alone to refer to infectious mononucleosis. [EU]

Mycobacterium: An organism of the genus Mycobacterium. [EU]

Naegleria: A free-living soil amoeba pathogenic to humans and animals. It occurs also in water and sewage. The most commonly found species in man is naegleri fowleri which is the pathogen for primary amebic meningoencephalitis in primates. [NIH]

Natamycin: Amphoteric macrolide antifungal antibiotic from Streptomyces natalensis or S. chattanoogensis. It is used for a variety of fungal infections, mainly topically. [NIH]

Nausea: An unpleasant sensation, vaguely referred to the epigastrium and abdomen, and often culminating in vomiting. [EU]

Neomycin: Antibiotic complex produced by Streptomyces fradiae. It is composed of neomycins A, B, and C. It acts by inhibiting translation during protein synthesis. [NIH]

Neonatal: Pertaining to the first four weeks after birth. [EU]

Neurologic: Pertaining to neurology or to the nervous system. [EU]

Neurology: A medical specialty concerned with the study of the structures, functions, and diseases of the nervous system. [NIH]

Neutrophil: Having an affinity for neutral dyes. [EU]

Norfloxacin: Quinoline-derived synthetic antibacterial agent with a very broad spectrum of action. Oral administration yields highly bactericidal plasma, tissue, and urine levels. Norfloxacin inhibits bacterial DNA-gyrase and is used in gastrointestinal, eye, and urinary infections. [NIH]

Ophthalmology: A surgical specialty concerned with the structure and function of the eye and the medical and surgical treatment of its defects and diseases. [NIH]

Orthopaedic: Pertaining to the correction of deformities of the musculoskeletal system; pertaining to orthopaedics. [EU]

Osmolarity: The concentration of osmotically active particles expressed in terms of osmoles of solute per litre of solution. [EU]

Parasitic: Pertaining to, of the nature of, or caused by a parasite. [EU]

Parenchyma: The essential elements of an organ; used in anatomical nomenclature as a general term to designate the functional elements of an organ, as distinguished from its framework, or stroma. [EU]

Parvovirus: A genus of the family parvoviridae, subfamily parvovirinae, infecting a variety of vertebrates including humans. Parvoviruses are responsible for a number of important diseases but also can be non-pathogenic in certain hosts. The type species is mice minute virus. [NIH]

Perinatal: Pertaining to or occurring in the period shortly before and after birth; variously defined as beginning with completion of the twentieth to twenty-eighth week of gestation and ending 7 to 28 days after birth. [EU]

Perioperative: Pertaining to the period extending from the time of hospitalization for surgery to the time of discharge. [EU]

Phagocytosis: Endocytosis of particulate material, such as microorganisms or cell fragments. The material is taken into the cell in membrane-bound vesicles (phagosomes) that originate as pinched off invaginations of the plasma membrane. Phagosomes fuse with lysosomes, forming phagolysosomes in which the engulfed material is killed and digested. [EU]

Pharyngitis: Inflammation of the pharynx. [EU]

Phenotype: The outward appearance of the individual. It is the product of interactions between genes and between the genotype and the environment. This includes the killer phenotype, characteristic of yeasts. [NIH]

Placenta: A highly vascular fetal organ through which the fetus absorbs oxygen and other nutrients and excretes carbon dioxide and other wastes. It begins to form about the eighth day of gestation when the blastocyst adheres to the decidua. [NIH]

Pneumonia: Inflammation of the lungs with consolidation. [EU]

Polymyxin: Basic polypeptide antibiotic group obtained from Bacillus polymyxa. They affect the cell membrane by detergent action and may cause neuromuscular and kidney damage. At least eleven different members of the polymyxin group have been identified, each designated by a letter. [NIH]

Postnatal: Occurring after birth, with reference to the newborn. [EU]

Prednisolone: A glucocorticoid with the general properties of the corticosteroids. It is the drug of choice for all conditions in which routine systemic corticosteroid therapy is indicated, except adrenal deficiency states. [NIH]

Prenatal: Existing or occurring before birth, with reference to the fetus. [EU]

Prevalence: The total number of cases of a given disease in a specified population at a designated time. It is differentiated from incidence, which refers to the number of new cases in the population at a given time. [NIH]

Prophylaxis: The prevention of disease; preventive treatment. [EU]

Proteins: Polymers of amino acids linked by peptide bonds. The specific sequence of amino acids determines the shape and function of the protein. [NIH]

Pseudomonas: A genus of gram-negative, aerobic, rod-shaped bacteria widely distributed in nature. Some species are pathogenic for humans, animals, and plants. [NIH]

Psychiatry: The medical science that deals with the origin, diagnosis, prevention, and treatment of mental disorders. [NIH]

Pulmonary: Pertaining to the lungs. [EU]

Receptor: 1. a molecular structure within a cell or on the surface characterized by (1) selective binding of a specific substance and (2) a specific physiologic effect that accompanies the binding, e.g., cell-surface receptors for peptide hormones, neurotransmitters, antigens, complement fragments, and immunoglobulins and cytoplasmic receptors for steroid hormones. 2. a sensory nerve terminal that responds to stimuli of various kinds. [EU]

Recombinant: 1. a cell or an individual with a new combination of genes not found together in either parent; usually applied to linked genes. [EU]

Recurrence: The return of a sign, symptom, or disease after a remission. [NIH]

Sarcoma: A tumour made up of a substance like the embryonic connective tissue; tissue composed of closely packed cells embedded in a fibrillar or homogeneous substance. Sarcomas are often highly malignant. [EU]

Schizophrenia: A severe emotional disorder of psychotic depth characteristically marked by a retreat from reality with delusion formation, hallucinations, emotional disharmony, and regressive behavior. [NIH]

Sclerosis: A induration, or hardening; especially hardening of a part from inflammation and in diseases of the interstitial substance. The term is used chiefly for such a hardening of the nervous system due to hyperplasia of the connective tissue or to designate hardening of the blood vessels. [EU]

Seizures: Clinical or subclinical disturbances of cortical function due to a sudden, abnormal, excessive, and disorganized discharge of brain cells. Clinical manifestations include abnormal motor, sensory and psychic phenomena. Recurrent seizures are usually referred to as epilepsy or "seizure disorder." [NIH]

Seroconversion: The change of a serologic test from negative to positive, indicating the development of antibodies in response to infection or immunization. [EU]

Serology: The study of serum, especially of antigen-antibody reactions in vitro. [NIH]

Species: A taxonomic category subordinate to a genus (or subgenus) and superior to a subspecies or variety, composed of individuals possessing common characters distinguishing them from other categories of individuals of the same taxonomic level. In taxonomic nomenclature, species are designated by the genus name followed by a Latin or Latinized adjective or noun. [EU]

Spermicide: An agent that is destructive to spermatozoa. [EU]

Spores: The reproductive elements of lower organisms, such as protozoa, fungi, and cryptogamic plants. [NIH]

Subacute: Somewhat acute; between acute and chronic. [EU]

Subarachnoid: Situated or occurring between the arachnoid and the pia mater. [EU]

Subclinical: Without clinical manifestations; said of the early stage(s) of an infection or other disease or abnormality before symptoms and signs become apparent or detectable by clinical examination or laboratory tests, or of a very mild form of an infection or other disease or abnormality. [EU]

Sulfadiazine: A short-acting sulfonamide used in combination with pyrimethamine to treat toxoplasmosis in patients with acquired immunodeficiency syndrome and in newborns with congenital infections. [NIH]

Superinfection: A new infection complicating the course of antimicrobial therapy of an existing infectious process, and resulting from invasion by bacteria or fungi resistant to the drug(s) in use. It may occur at the site of the original infection or at a remote site. [EU]

Symptomatic: 1. pertaining to or of the nature of a symptom. 2. indicative (of a particular disease or disorder). 3. exhibiting the symptoms of a particular disease but having a different cause. 4. directed at the allying of symptoms, as symptomatic treatment. [EU]

Systemic: Pertaining to or affecting the body as a whole. [EU]

Tetanus: A disease caused by tetanospasmin, a powerful protein toxin produced by clostridium tetani. Tetanus usually occurs after an acute injury, such as a puncture wound or laceration. Generalized tetanus, the most common form, is characterized by tetanic muscular contractions and hyperreflexia. Localized tetanus presents itself as a mild condition with manifestations restricted to muscles near the wound. It may progress to the generalized form. [NIH]

Tobramycin: An aminoglycoside, broad-spectrum antibiotic produced by Streptomyces tenebrarius. It is effective against gram-negative bacteria, especially the Pseudomonas species. It is a 10% component of the antibiotic complex, nebramycin, produced by the same species. [NIH]

Tolerance: 1. the ability to endure unusually large doses of a drug or toxin. 2. acquired drug tolerance; a decreasing response to repeated constant doses of a drug or the need for increasing doses to maintain a constant response. [EU]

Topical: Pertaining to a particular surface area, as a topical anti-infective applied to a certain area of the skin and affecting only the area to which it is applied. [EU]

Toxicology: The science concerned with the detection, chemical composition, and pharmacologic action of toxic substances or poisons and the treatment and prevention of toxic manifestations. [NIH]

Transplantation: The grafting of tissues taken from the patient's own body or from another. [EU]

Tuberculosis: Any of the infectious diseases of man and other animals caused by species of mycobacterium. [NIH]

Ulcer: A local defect, or excavation, of the surface of an organ or tissue; which is produced by the sloughing of inflammatory necrotic tissue. [EU]

Urinary: Pertaining to the urine; containing or secreting urine. [EU]

Vaccine: A suspension of attenuated or killed microorganisms (bacteria, viruses, or rickettsiae), administered for the prevention, amelioration or treatment of infectious diseases. [EU]

Vaginal: 1. of the nature of a sheath; ensheathing. 2. pertaining to the vagina. 3. pertaining to the tunica vaginalis testis. [EU]

Venereal: Pertaining or related to or transmitted by sexual contact. [EU]

Ventilation: 1. in respiratory physiology, the process of exchange of air between the lungs and the ambient air. Pulmonary ventilation (usually measured in litres per minute) refers to the total exchange, whereas alveolar ventilation refers to the effective ventilation of the alveoli, in which gas exchange with the blood takes place. 2. in psychiatry, verbalization of one's emotional problems. [EU]

Viral: Pertaining to, caused by, or of the nature of virus. [EU]

Viremia: The presence of viruses in the blood. [NIH]

Virion: The infective system of a virus, composed of the viral genome, a protein core, and a protein coat called a capsid, which may be naked or enclosed in a lipoprotein envelope called the peplos. [NIH]

Warts: Benign epidermal proliferations or tumors; some are viral in origin. [NIH]

General Dictionaries and Glossaries

While the above glossary is essentially complete, the dictionaries listed here cover virtually all aspects of medicine, from basic words and phrases to more advanced terms (sorted alphabetically by title; hyperlinks provide rankings, information and reviews at Amazon.com):

- **Dictionary of Medical Acronymns & Abbreviations** by Stanley Jablonski (Editor), Paperback, 4th edition (2001), Lippincott Williams & Wilkins Publishers, ISBN: 1560534605, http://www.amazon.com/exec/obidos/ASIN/1560534605/icongroupinterna

- **Dictionary of Medical Terms : For the Nonmedical Person (Dictionary of Medical Terms for the Nonmedical Person, Ed 4)** by Mikel A. Rothenberg, M.D, et al, Paperback - 544 pages, 4th edition (2000), Barrons Educational Series, ISBN: 0764112015, http://www.amazon.com/exec/obidos/ASIN/0764112015/icongroupinterna

- **A Dictionary of the History of Medicine** by A. Sebastian, CD-Rom edition (2001), CRC Press-Parthenon Publishers, ISBN: 185070368X, http://www.amazon.com/exec/obidos/ASIN/185070368X/icongroupinterna

- **Dorland's Illustrated Medical Dictionary (Standard Version)** by Dorland, et al, Hardcover - 2088 pages, 29th edition (2000), W B Saunders Co, ISBN: 0721662544, http://www.amazon.com/exec/obidos/ASIN/0721662544/icongroupinterna

- **Dorland's Electronic Medical Dictionary** by Dorland, et al, Software, 29th Book & CD-Rom edition (2000), Harcourt Health Sciences, ISBN: 0721694934, http://www.amazon.com/exec/obidos/ASIN/0721694934/icongroupinterna

- **Dorland's Pocket Medical Dictionary (Dorland's Pocket Medical Dictionary, 26th Ed)** Hardcover - 912 pages, 26th edition (2001), W B Saunders Co, ISBN: 0721682812, http://www.amazon.com/exec/obidos/ASIN/0721682812/icongroupinterna /103-4193558-7304618

- **Melloni's Illustrated Medical Dictionary (Melloni's Illustrated Medical Dictionary, 4th Ed)** by Melloni, Hardcover, 4th edition (2001), CRC Press-Parthenon Publishers, ISBN: 85070094X, http://www.amazon.com/exec/obidos/ASIN/85070094X/icongroupinterna

- **Stedman's Electronic Medical Dictionary Version 5.0 (CD-ROM for Windows and Macintosh, Individual)** by Stedmans, CD-ROM edition (2000), Lippincott Williams & Wilkins Publishers, ISBN: 0781726328, http://www.amazon.com/exec/obidos/ASIN/0781726328/icongroupinterna

- **Stedman's Medical Dictionary** by Thomas Lathrop Stedman, Hardcover - 2098 pages, 27th edition (2000), Lippincott, Williams & Wilkins, ISBN: 068340007X,
  http://www.amazon.com/exec/obidos/ASIN/068340007X/icongroupinterna

- **Tabers Cyclopedic Medical Dictionary (Thumb Index)** by Donald Venes (Editor), et al, Hardcover - 2439 pages, 19th edition (2001), F A Davis Co, ISBN: 0803606540,
  http://www.amazon.com/exec/obidos/ASIN/0803606540/icongroupinterna

INDEX

Printed in the United States
60096LVS00005B/32